SHEAR FORCE

An image-maker's memoir

Allen Edwards

with

Lorin Shields-Michel

Durban House

Printed in the United States of America.

For information address:

Durban House Publishing Company, Inc.
7502 Greenville Avenue, Suite 500, Dallas, Texas 75231

Library of Congress Cataloging-in-Publication Data

Edwards, Allen, and Shields-Michel, Lorin

Shear Force / Allen Edwards and Lorin Shields-Michel

Library of Congress Control Number: 2008931919

p. cm.

ISBN: 978-0-9779863-6-1

First Edition

10 9 8 7 6 5 4 3 2 1

Visit our Web site at
http://www.durbanhouse.com

For Lisa

Amy, Jason, Megan and Samantha

and my grandchildren

Benny, Jacob and Ethan

Table of Contents

Introduction

1989

"You're losing it." As my lawyer said the words I could see them hanging in the air like a dialogue balloon from a cartoon. "The Beverly Hills salon—well, you can't afford it. You've got a $1 million lease and no hairdressers. You've got Irvine and Woodland Hills, plus two others. I don't see how you can stay in Beverly Hills. You're hemorrhaging hairdressers, you've got no staff."

He paused. Then went for the jugular: "Allen. Either you lose it or you sell it."

I sat in the chair behind my desk, my back ramrod straight. My head was spinning. It hurt. The business I'd spent so many years building up, the reputation I had painstakingly formulated, my precious Beverly Hills, the crème de la crème of locations, was in flames. All because my partner, after 20 years, had decided he didn't want to cut hair anymore. He'd rather play golf and hang out with his stockbroker. He'd been sucking the business dry with his salary while I worked my ass off. I had decided to split off from him, and now that decision was hanging over me like Death with his sickle poised to cut off my head, or some other equally arrogant part of my body. My staff. My hairdressers. Gone. All of it gone, or close to it. Nothing left. I was down to my last few dollars. I actually thought about pulling out my wallet just then, if for no other reason than to show that it wasn't all gone. I had at least a twenty.

But if I didn't close Beverly Hills, would I be broke? Yes. According to my lawyer, if I didn't close Beverly Hills, I'd go bankrupt. I knew nothing about bankruptcy. What did it mean? Would I lose everything?

This was where my survival instincts kicked in. I was Rambo with a blow dryer.

Don't procrastinate. Make a move. Get off your ass and do something. Anything.

My mind was reeling. I could almost hear my brain spinning.

I did have other salons. They were doing well, OK. Newport, Irvine, Long Beach. Sure, I'd given my partner Encino so that I could keep Beverly Hills. But still, how could I be losing it? How?

My wife, Lisa, and I had talked about this. Beverly Hills had been jamming, and now all of a sudden it was gone. It was like being blind-sided… I had gotten rid of Paul, my partner, because I knew that I could do it on my own. That, and he just plain pissed me off. I had given him the Encino salon as part of the deal. But now Beverly Hills was worthless, it had a million-dollar lease, and all I could think was, "I have nothing. My empire's crumbling and Paul's got a new salon in Encino."

"You're going to have to give it all up, Allen."

It hit me then. I was about to become everything that I had vowed I would never be. Like my father before me, who never achieved the success that I'm sure he dreamed of, I felt like a failure. My father's face passed before my eyes. It was a tired, ragged face. Kind, but disappointed. Worn down by the years and lack of drive and desire to truly change his life.

He was a good father, my father, always there for us. Still, he never really amounted to anything more than a middle-class worker. There's nothing wrong with that, of course; I just wanted more. When he was young he was a singer and a dancer, but he never pursued it. His mother told him, "It's not a good career; you'll never amount to anything." And he didn't, not really. He lived his sad life, working for a laundry service that sold towels and uniforms to garages and gas stations. He had a nagging wife. I had vowed I would never live like that and would always follow whatever my dream was, and my dream was to be a famous hairdresser.

When I was a kid, I had loved the smell of oil and the garage. I loved stopping with my dad at greasy spoons and eating French dip sandwiches and fries. I loved being on the road. It's amazing I didn't want to become a truck driver. I remember meeting the big boss. And I knew that's who I wanted to be. Not my dad. I wanted to make the rules, not follow them. I would be successful.

I would rock the world.

Now here I was, sitting in my office. I could smell the fragrance of the salon, shampoos and hairspray co-mingling with the chemicals of perms and color. I could hear the silence, the deafening silence of the missing hairdressers and their clients. I still dream about having empty salons and no hairdressers.

You're going to have to give it all up, Allen.

"No, I-I-I-I." I stopped.

I had stuttered as a kid. It came back to me occasionally in adulthood, when I was faced with a situation over which I felt I had no control. *You're. Giving. Up.* I was becoming the loser I was afraid of being.

"I'm not," I said.

My lawyer looked at me with a quizzical look.

"I'm not giving it up," I said.

And then I smiled.

"You know what? Fuck it. I've still got my name."

I'm Rambo. With a blow dryer.

one

I Was a Teenage Stutterer

"Hey, nice hair." The kid was good-looking, dressed in the style of the day. Probably jeans and a button down shirt, but I don't remember now. I didn't know his name. I didn't say anything.

The guy looked at me for a long minute.

"What's your name?" he asked.

Still, I said nothing.

"Well, OK. See ya around," he said, shrugging his shoulders and leaving with his friends, all of them dressed in jeans with big cuffs, white bucks, a cardigan sweater.

I stood there watching them go. I wanted to shout "ALLEN!" Hell, I just wanted to say "Allen," but nothing would come out of my mouth. I was new at school—we'd just moved from Hollywood to Canoga Park—and I stood there, at Canoga Park High, watching the cool kids, who should have been my friends immediately because I had the look, the hair, the walk, but I didn't have the talk.

In junior high, in Hollywood, where I grew up, I had millions of friends (OK, an exaggeration, but I had a lot), I was first trumpet in the band, I had a reputation for being a great dancer. I was Mister Popular, and now, I was at a new school where nobody knew anything about me. I was like Kevin Bacon in the movie *Footloose*, with the looks, the hair, the dancing. Only he didn't stutter. My situation was worse.

Fact was, I wanted to tell him, tell them all, what my name was, but I couldn't get the words out. I stuttered. Not the kind of stuttering where a person stammers. I stuttered by opening my mouth and having the words get caught in the back of my throat where they choked me half to death every time I was faced with a situation where I was uncomfortable, which was damned close to every day at school, especially after my family moved to Canoga Park in the San Fernando Valley when I was in high school.

It was humiliating. I knew I had to get over it.

I had some speech therapy in school, but that didn't help me. At the time, no one went to any other kind of therapy. I had to find a way to get comfortable. When I was comfortable in a situation, I was OK. I could talk.

So I stood there, my first day of high school, watching all the kids. The sweaters were all green, the school color. A lot of them had letters, really big letters. And I wanted that. I had to have the big letterman sweater. I had the look, but I had to have the sweater. I was into fashion, and if green letter sweaters were the fashion, then that's what I needed. Funny thing is, years later, before I graduated, I finally did letter. In band. (Please. Band?) Not exactly cool.

I remember thinking, "How did it come to this?"

I was born in Chicago on January 3, 1945, the second child of Sam and Betty Goldstein. My sister Ros, short for Roslyn, was eight when I made my appearance. My brother Jerry entered the picture five years later. He stuttered, too. We lived in Chicago for only a short time before moving to Hollywood. I was one at the time. We had a nice little house, right in front of my grandparents'. I loved Hollywood. It was easy. And even though I had problems talking sometimes, it didn't matter as much. It wouldn't matter until I got older, until Canoga Park.

I went to Vine Street Grammar School, where the kids were tough. They actually looked like some of the older kids, like in the movie *Grease.* Black leather jackets, motorcycle boots and big, thick belts with the buckle pulled over to the side. The daily chores were to try to kiss a girl, not get beat up, and get through class without having to talk.

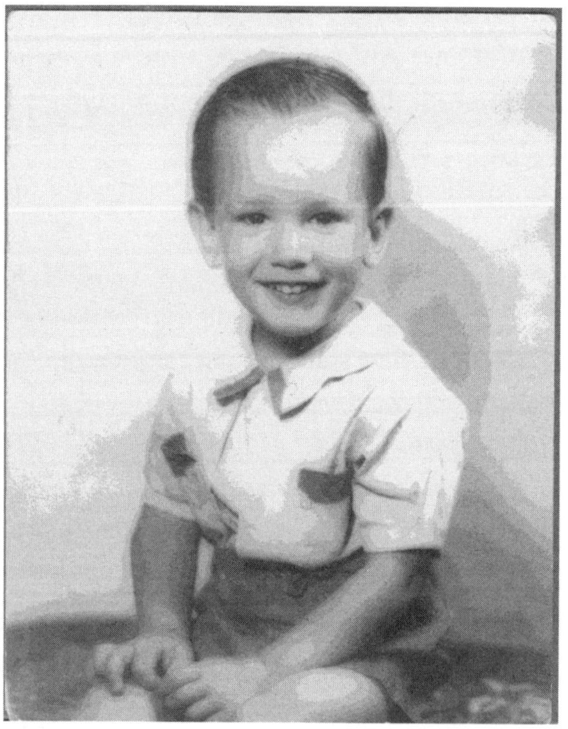

Me.

We were typical middle class, with working cars and a decent house. My grandfather owned the property. He also had one eye and was missing three fingers. I never did find out why. We put a house on his lot, right at Gower and Romaine, by the studios. My father had actually bought a house in Westchester, and they moved the house on a truck, in pieces, to the lot. I didn't know you could do that.

It was the early 1950s and the world was sort of black and white. The war was over, but society hadn't decided what it wanted to be yet. It had a true air of innocence. We played baseball on the lawn at Gower Cemetery and we toured the world on customized bikes with ape handlebars and cut-off fenders. There were bullies and tough guys all around us, and nobody with any money. A hooker lived next door. Across the street was a '57 Cadillac convertible owned by Mrs. Dunson, who used to run around the house in a mink coat, completely naked underneath. (Wonder where she is now?) I didn't know her first name. Her older daughter was Michelle, and we used to make out all the time. During the '50s, with not much else going on, we made out so much, it's amazing our lips didn't fall off. I'm not sure that I knew how to French kiss until the middle of 7th grade. That's when I learned to use my tongue. The first time I French kissed, I thought I was going to catch some wild disease. I ran home and told my mother, who actually laughed.

"It's just part of kissing," she said.

That gave me a green light as far as I was concerned to go and make out with everyone, and to become an expert with my tongue. I think at some point I actually had fantasies about Michelle's mother. Sometimes I think I actually still do. (But only when I need it.) It was always a fantasy to be seduced by my girlfriend's mother. My fantasy was this: she would put on her makeup, she would call me into her room, and her fur coat would be open and she would make me do nasty things to her while she was applying her makeup (I was always into fashion… and Avon).

She was the hottest woman I'd ever seen. I was young.

Hollywood in those days was a different kind of stimulating than it is today. The air was cleaner and the streets were dirtier. I remember walking down Gower, toward the Boulevard, and letting the town sort of wash over me, like a cool splash from a standing puddle. The smells were fried chicken and eucalyptus, intermingling in the air and in my nose. Birds would whistle in the trees, a car would backfire, and I felt like I was living the life that Don McLean eventually sang about in "American Pie." I was the typical "American Pie" guy, though I wouldn't realize that until the song was released years later, in October of 1971. There was something about the lyrics, the longing for a different time, that haunted me. Music did make me smile; I did love to dance.

I was always interested in the kids on TV, in the dancing, the music on *American Bandstand*, and of course, the girls. I also used to fantasize about being one of the guys on *American Bandstand* in the suit and tie and dance on the bandstand. Of course, I also wanted to be a Mouseketeer and French kiss Annette. My fear, though, was that I would have to say my name and I couldn't get it out. How could I be a Mouseketeer if I couldn't say my name at the beginning?

These two guys that I remember—Bobby Cohn and Bruce Booker—they were tough guys, and that intrigued me, too. But when I was young, I wasn't tough enough or brave enough to be like them. (I wonder where they are today. Are they lawyers or are they in prison?) The first vision of cool that I really remember was my friend Jimmy Beavers' brother. He was driving a 1950 Panhead Harley with ape-hangers, had a jellyroll haircut and his cigarettes rolled in his sleeve. That was an amazing sight to me as a kid. Bobby and Bruce were the tough guys of the school and only interested in beating people up.

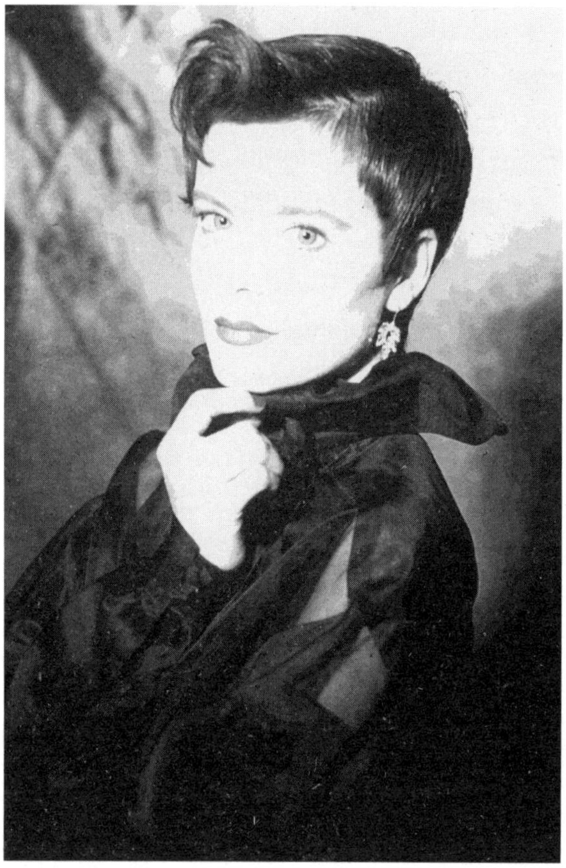

Years later, I recreated the '50s look on my stage models.

"Hey, kid," they'd call. I don't know which one called it. They were inseparable and identical in their black leather jackets.

"We got nothin' to do today. Thought we'd punch the stutterer."

They'd laugh at me, sneer and punch me in the stomach or the arm. It didn't matter. It always hurt. I actually ended up fighting with them about once a week. I wasn't afraid to fight back, and they had a grudging respect for me because I wasn't afraid of them. I took my aggression out on another kid named Donald Maxfield. He was the school cello player (I think he was gay, not that there's anything wrong with that) and the cello just wasn't cool. I'd knock him down, knock the wind out of him, and I'd feel good. I played the trumpet, starting when I was eight. It felt cold and sleek in my hand. Sexy. And I was good at it. I also discovered something interesting: when you're good at something, people learn to respect you for your talents instead of harassing you about your weaknesses. For some stupid reason, people who stutter are perceived as stupid or a "retard," to put it in kid-speak, which isn't the case at all. Stutterers just can't talk.

Stuttering is actually a complex set of behaviors that happen at once in the brain. Sometimes it involves repeating sounds, syllables or words (th-the-the). It can also involve a prolonged silence where the mouth is open and no sound is coming out. The exact cause of stuttering isn't known yet, but there are three theories. The leading theory says that stuttering is a learned behavior. A second theory says that it's a psychological problem that can be treated with therapy. A third theory states that stuttering is organic, that neurological differences exist between the brains of those who stutter and those who don't. Although the interference with speaking can be triggered by emotional or situational factors (like being challenged at school), stuttering is not psychological. People who stutter are completely and perfectly normal in all other aspects of their lives. Except the talking part.

Imagine someone coming up to you and you can't get words out.

"What's a matter? Don't you know your name?"

It's an icy, cold feeling that flows through your body, followed by dead panic. So you start practicing because you know what someone is going to ask you, and you still can't get it out. It's like being in a play and you rehearse and rehearse and rehearse because you've got one line but it's a really important line. Opening night comes, you've got the line down pat, and then you're in front of the audience and it's your turn to speak. And nothing. It's gone. There's nothing in your head. That's the panic. Everyone has experienced this at one time or another. I experienced it daily.

Funny thing was, I didn't stutter when I chose to talk. In fact, most stutterers don't stutter when they sing, or act, or when they play a musical instrument.

And I loved to talk. I wanted to talk. Talking eventually made me famous. Go figure. But back then, I couldn't. At least, I couldn't until I found the trumpet. Somehow that musical instrument, with its soulful notes, allowed me to speak normally. I'd have these fantasies (always with the fantasies), where someone would come up to me and ask me something as simple as...

"What's your name, kid?"

And I'd answer, speaking as if I were using my fingers, playing the trumpet. I'd answer with a blow of the horn. I could carry on an entire conversation using my trumpet.

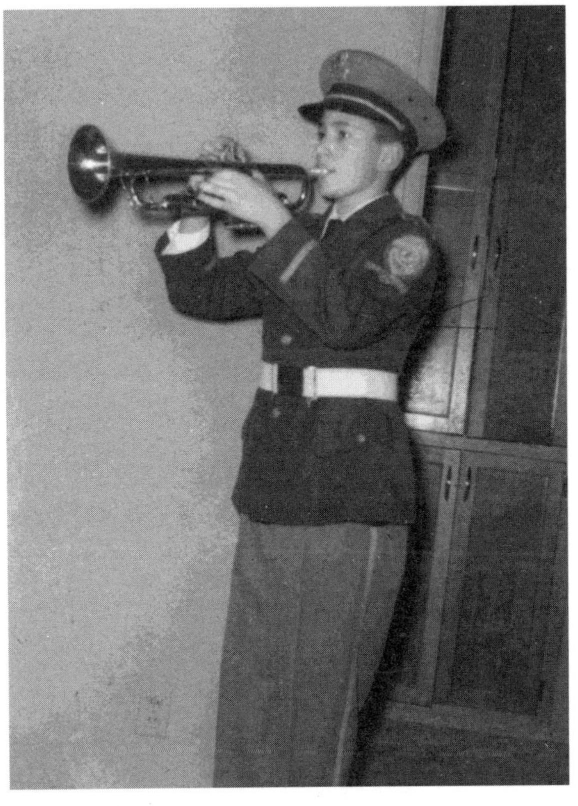

Communicating without a stutter, through my trumpet.

"Toot." Translation: Allen.

"Play any sports?"

"Roa Waa." Translation: a little baseball. A little basketball.

"Great. Suit up."

"Waa waa toot soallll." Translation: I'm ready!

I stuttered. So what?

I had to be the best, best, best. It was a cover-up for my stuttering. I was never the last one chosen when teams were suiting up. I was always up there in the sports category. I was the best dancer in school. I was first trumpet in the band.

When I started junior high at Lacont Junior High, in Hollywood, some of the kids made fun of me, but I was getting cute, so the girls liked me and that made me fit in. I also found that I liked rich kids. There was one girl, Diane Mecklenberg, a short Jewish girl with glasses and curly hair,

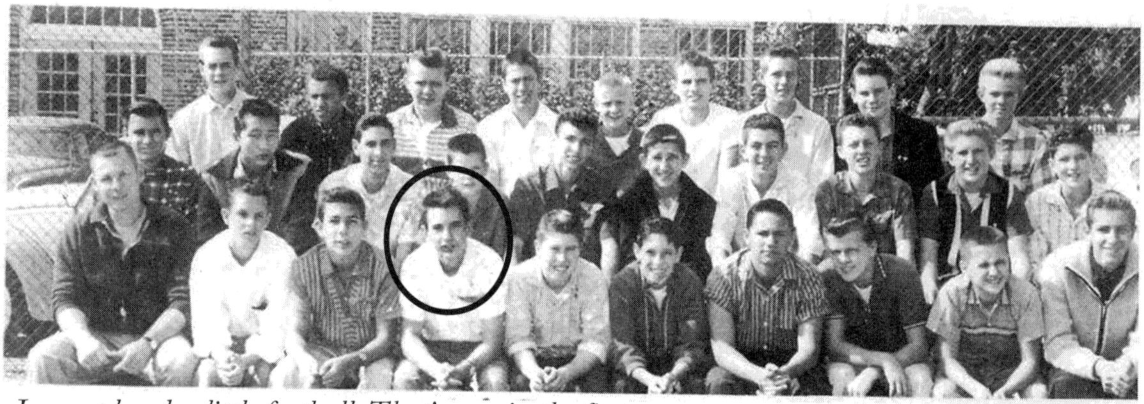

I even played a little football. That's me, in the first row.

who lived in this huge house in Los Feliz. She was my first girlfriend and she helped me to gain some confidence. She had braces. It kind of turned me on. (I'm still trying to figure that out.)

Roger, my best friend from grammar school, suddenly wasn't cool enough for me anymore. I developed a new group of friends, Joel and Dwayne, and I fit in with the more popular, richer kids. I didn't hang out with kids from the neighborhood anymore. I started to think maybe I had just been born into the wrong family. (Where are my real parents anyway? Isn't my dad somebody like Donald Trump?) I felt more comfortable around more successful people.

Being in the popular group also meant I wasn't getting beat up as much. In fact, I was excelling. I found out that I liked to be the performer. I ran for office and got elected VP of the student council. "Be a pal, vote for Al." That was my campaign slogan. When I ran for office, I didn't stutter. But when I had to give up my chair to the person who would take my place, I stuttered. Go figure. It's hard to let go of fame.

There were talent shows. First place, first year. Second place, second year. I was never afraid to get into anything, even though I stuttered. I tried to ignore it, as much as I could anyway. I helped set up dances at school. I played spin the bottle and post office. (I loved making out. Too bad I couldn't get a job being a professional kisser.) Those were the big games of the time. Nobody got hurt. It was an innocent time, when there were only sports, girls and cars.

Still, many mornings I'd wake up in a cold sweat. I was popular, but the fear of stuttering was overwhelming. There's nothing like the terror of knowing that if someone talks to you, nothing will come out of your own mouth but hot breath. Nothing like it, especially when you're young. You know if you can't get the words out, your face will contort as you try to do anything you can to get them out. Society finds stuttering funny, so they laugh at stutterers. But there's nothing funny about it when it's happening to you. I was terrified of having to get up in class to speak, of reading from a book when called on. I would sit in the back of the classroom and watch the clock, counting the number of

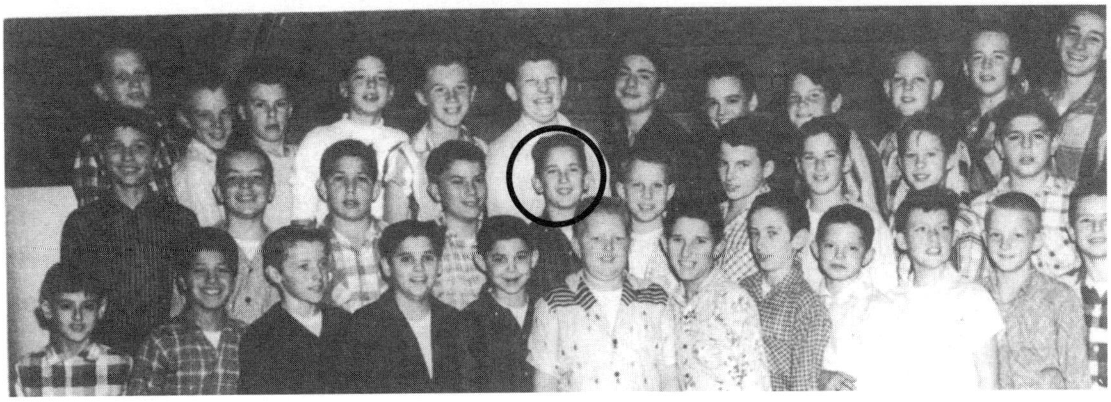

I really hated school.

people the teacher would have to go through before he got to me. I wanted to vomit. Sometimes I did.

Then we moved to Canoga Park. Life ended.

In those days, in the late '50s, early '60s, Canoga Park was a pretty place. There were lots of trees, lots of houses, and lots of clean air. The Valley hadn't been exploited yet. The developers hadn't gotten hold of it. It was still nice, sweet, with orange trees. I hated it.

I missed hitchhiking down Vine Street to go to the movies. I missed my hooker next door. I missed making out with my neighbor. I was stuck in a little house, lonely and having nothing to look forward to but the first day of school.

Holy shit.

I wore my black tanker jacket, white t-shirt and Levi's. I tried to look cool. But every time someone asked me my name, it took me four minutes to get the words out. Four minutes. That's longer than it takes some people to run a mile.

At first, I ate lunch by myself and all the nerds and dopes eventually became my friends. One of my biggest problems was that there were no rich kids. I felt comfortable with the rich, not the farmers. I was in the band, probably the only place I still felt good about myself, still clinging to my beloved trumpet. I was 2nd trumpet at CP High. First trumpet was a senior named Mike Baromen who looked like he was 50. He was the only kid who walked around in a corduroy sports coat carrying his trumpet. He had nerd written all over him. Every time I'd miss a note, he'd hit me (on the leg) as hard as he could. He was into his man thing. I was a freshman. He was a senior. I hated him. But I also admired him and wanted to be better than him.

The interesting thing about band was that all people in the band were nice because in those days, we were all hated together. We were hated for our outfits and our plumes. I was also the only Jew in the whole school, or so I thought. I started hanging out with the AZA, a Jewish boys' group in the area. Most of the Jewish kids went to Birmingham High in Encino. They had money. Hooray. I liked them. They weren't focused only on wearing green cardigan sweaters with giant C letters. We liked to meet up with the BBG girls' group. Things started to get better. My stutter started to go away as I felt more comfortable with what I was doing. I liked the girls at Birmingham High.

I became first trumpet when Mike left. I also got the responsibility to do bugle call in the morning. Nerd. I decided to change the way the band played. I raised the music an octave and started playing more big band stuff. I started going to the dances, and I started to shine in the girls' eyes. They noticed me. The athletes couldn't do anything but stumble on the dance floor. Now they were in my territory. I was the performer. I was hot again. But I never truly fit in. I was like the cool peg in the nerd hole.

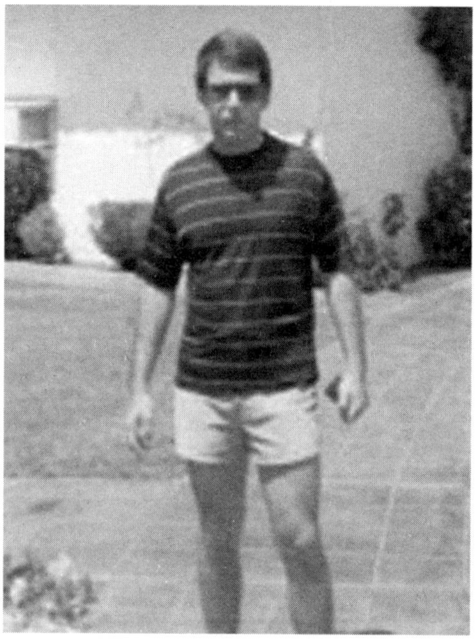

Nerd.

In my sophomore year I was voted best dressed. Go figure, I thought they all hated me. I was in.

My confidence soared, except when it didn't. I was a b-b-b-basketball player, and my stuttering would once again rear its ugly little monster head every time I'd have to tell the announcer that I was subbing for someone.

G-g-g-g-g-g-g-g-oldstein for Smith.

The anxiety would take all the energy and air right out of me.

At home, things were what I thought was normal for a family of five. A weak father, a dominating mother, an older sister with anxiety problems and a younger brother also cursed with stuttering. The great American Jewish family. We never talked about any of that. There was no mention of Ros' anxiety or my stuttering or Jerry's stuttering.

My goal was to not be my father, and I carried this little Allen around on my shoulder, constantly telling me, "You're going to be just like him. You're not going to make it; you'll never amount to anything." Always negative, and all because I stuttered. But I eventually killed little Allen. Life got better.

I started dating a girl named Midge who went to Van Nuys High. She was 5' tall, Jewish, middle class, with a father who sold Fuller brushes. He was a "Fuller brush man." He was very much like my dad, though I really liked him. Midge's dad actually gave me one of my first jobs, delivering the Fuller brushes.

I bought my first car, a 1952 Ford convertible, for $300, and I thought I was in my blue heaven, which I actually wrote on the back of my continental kit. Maybe I was a nerd. In shop in school, I made a metal thumb for the gearshift knob. How cool was that? Only I thought so. (Oh. My. God. I *am* a nerd.) I crawled under the car and made holes in the muffler so it would sound big and bad.

I wanted to be accepted. I started dressing different to be popular. I had lettered in band (more nerd confirmation). But there was no way I was going to wear a letterman sweater with a C and a plume for band. Might as well have been an L for loser. That's when I decided I needed to change my look. I chose… surfer. (Yeah, that's it. I'll look like a surfer.) I bleached the front of my hair blonde, wore khakis, Pendleton shirts and black tennis shoes. I didn't surf, of course; Jews don't surf. The water is too cold. I was actually what they called a grimy, a make-believe surfer. All the surfers drove Woodies and were in their own world. But I hung out at the beach for the girls. For fun, we used to flip bottle caps at them. Picture five little Jews—Allen and his posse—at State Beach, sitting against the wall, flipping bottle caps. No wonder I couldn't get a date.

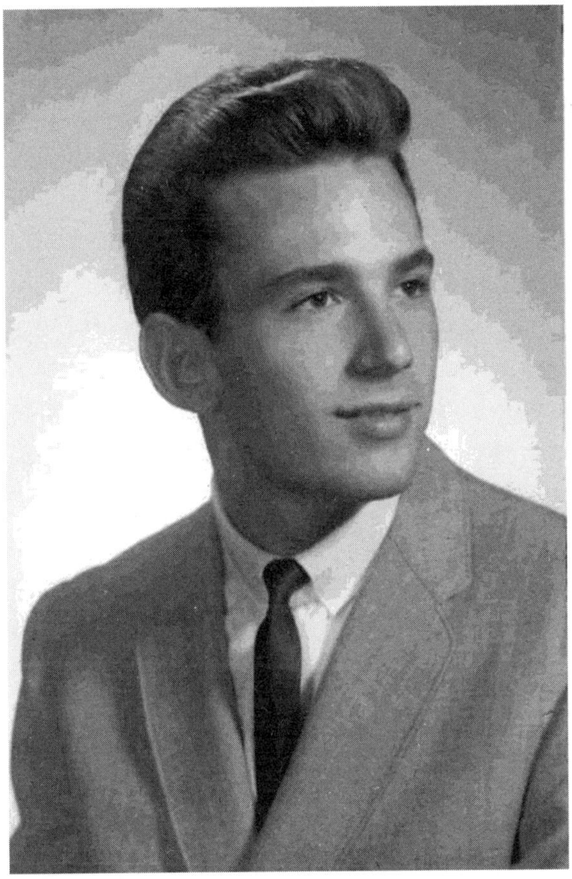

My yearbook picture. I looked like Bobby Darin.

Then it was 1963 and time for graduation. I was asked to play a solo, so I played a piece by Brahms. It was four pages, and it was just my trumpet and me. And an 18-piece band. I finally became the star of my class. I wanted them to hear me play. I wanted them to hear the music coming from my horn and know that I was speaking to them. I was saying "fuck you, fuck you, fuck you." I wanted them to know how happy I was to finally be getting away from the pressure. I was done with high school, and I'd never been so happy in my life.

Armed with my trumpet, my drive to not be my father, and my desire to stop stuttering once and for all, I went back to Hollywood. I bought a fake ID and started going to clubs, like the Chez Paris on Fairfax in Los Angeles, a very ethnically mixed club. Dancers had no color. I started dating Beverly, a black girl (taboo in those days), and had a buddy named Clifford with a gold tooth who was a phenomenal dancer. The girls had the biggest hair I'd ever seen. Great bodies, kick-ass gorgeous in tight pants with stirrups.

One night, Cliff and I decided to go to Pomona to the Cinnamon Cinder and show how great we were. We danced the twist, the pony, the jerk, the shag, the hitchhike and the mashed potato. But Pomona, back then, wasn't real fond of blacks or Jews. It was like being at a Klan reunion. When they circled us at the club, it wasn't to applaud. We got out of there. Quick.

Eventually Beverly and I broke up. I took her home to meet my grandmother and mother, who were in the middle of a Bene Brith meeting with all of their Jewish friends. My mother quickly ushered us into the back room and threw us out the back door. She wasn't a racist, she just didn't get it. Ignorance soared in the early 1960s. After a month, Bev and I called it quits. It was time to move on. I needed to experience more women.

There was another Cinnamon Cinder in Studio City, owned by Bob Eubanks. The guy who parked cars there was Jon Peters. I didn't really know him then. It was much later that he and I would work together. I hooked up with guys from New York, France, Philly. I was stuck in the world between orgies and Passover. It was amazing.

I met one of the famed Mouseketeers, Cubby O'Brien, one of the guys I so desperately wanted to be when I was young. There was also an actor called Bobby Diamond who starred in a television show called *Fury*, about a black stallion. I hung out at Valley Junior College and took some classes. I was going to be a famous musician and dancer. I was in the dance band with musicians who were better than me. They weren't making a dime. I dropped out of school and quit playing trumpet.

And I started to worry: am I becoming my father?

The interesting thing was, during this time, my stuttering virtually disappeared. I didn't have to talk except when I chose to. I had to dance, and in the dance world, nobody cared what you sounded like, only that you could move.

I joined a fraternity. Pledges needed to bang on the door and shout out their name in order to get in. I couldn't ever get my name out. It got so bad that when they heard the silence, they'd let me in. They knew it was silent Al.

During one of the pledge meetings, I learned one of my biggest life lessons. There was this guy who had a parrot on his shoulder. It shit on him. All the pledges laughed and he said, "What are you laughing at? I've been shit on before." Lesson? Don't buy a parrot. Except I did buy one later on. And he did crap all over me. What the hell do I know?

I eventually quit the fraternity, too. It seemed I was quitting everything.

Then it hit me. Holy shit. "I'm 18 years old. What am I going to do now?"

I thought about being a professional dancer. Bobby Banus was an instructor and I walked into this studio, a very professional class full of girls and gay men. It was my first experience with gay people. It overwhelmed me. It scared me to death. I was sure they all wanted me because I was so damned cute.

My best friend at the time was a guy named Norman Block, this fast-talking, slick guy who was working to be a hairdresser.

Hairdresser.

That's like fashion, right?

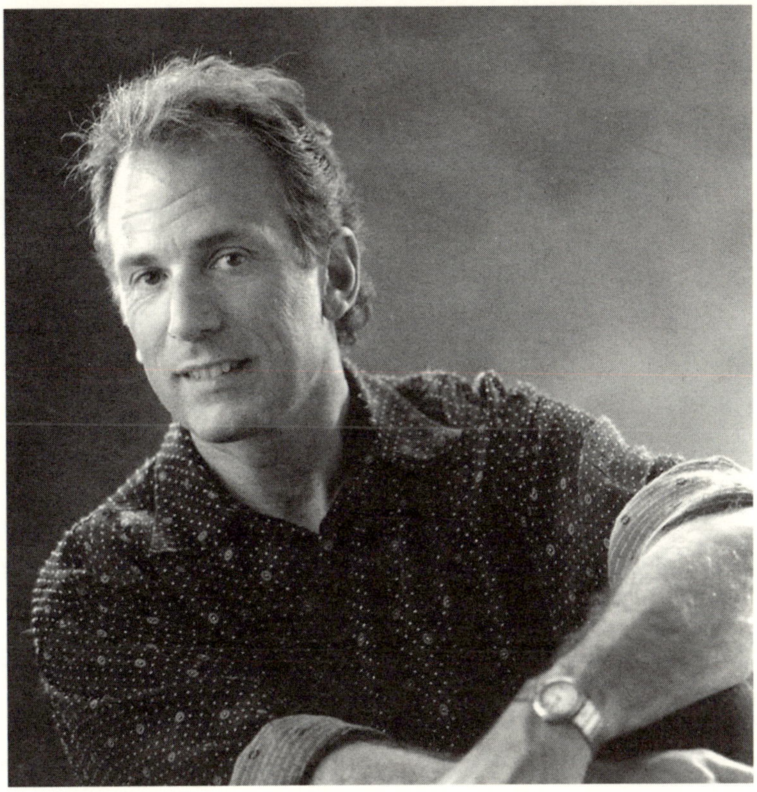

Allen Edwards

12

Hairdresser. That's like fashion, right?

two

Stories from the Beginning

Becoming a hairdresser

At 18, my whole life was already planned. I was going to play in a band, teach a little trumpet on the side, maybe even teach school. The problem was I was horrible at school unless it was a music course. At Valley Community College I found out something very important: I had to have a goal. But once I quit school and quit playing the trumpet, I didn't have a goal anymore. So I found myself doing a lot of nothing, horrible jobs.

I teamed up with two ex-convicts. It would have been better to have stayed in the gay dance class. I don't remember what they were in for. Probably stealing cars or old ladies' purses. We got this horse and we'd trot the horse into poor Spanish neighborhoods to convince the Hispanics to take pictures of their kids on the horse. Once again, I couldn't talk. The convicts took advantage of me and made me clean up after the horse, but at least they weren't staring at my ass. (Or maybe they were; they were in prison, after all.) I don't know how much money they made or when the horse finally died, but I quit that job pretty quickly because I had another really good job.

I cleaned pots and pans in a pizza place. But as I'd stand there with dirty, soapy, greasy water up to my elbows, I'd find myself thinking about when I used to deliver hair brushes door to door for Midge's father, the Fuller Brush man. I used to have this fantasy that some housewife would answer the door totally naked and lure me in. (I actually still have that fantasy.) Of course, once I got inside, all I'd get were cookies and a dog bite.

Hairdressing school was always in the back of my mind. I think someone came to high school once and talked about it. I thought about it, a lot.

After the pizza place, I got a job with the Tandy Leather Company. They sold leather goods to hospitals, as well as purses and dog collars. Very interesting combination. The office was in downtown Los Angeles, so whenever I was at the office, I'd find myself some female companionship in a poor tenement on 6th Street and Alvarado.

At night I'd dance until at least three. Get up early, go to work. But I was always sending things to the wrong hospitals because I was so tired from partying all night. Whenever anyone would yell at me, I would try to say something, but of course, I couldn't. One day, the owner was yelling at me about something. I told him to go fuck himself and decided right then and there to go to beauty school.

"Norm?" I said when Norman Block, my fast-talking buddy, answered his phone.

"Hey, A! How's the leather biz?" he asked. I could hear him sipping on a beer.

"I quit."

"Good for you," he said. "It was never really what you were meant for anyway."

Very prescient, that Norm.

"I was thinking," I said.

"Workin' without tools again, huh?" he said, laughing. Norman was always talking over me and laughing. But he was a good guy and he was my friend.

"I was thinking about Yamanos," I said.

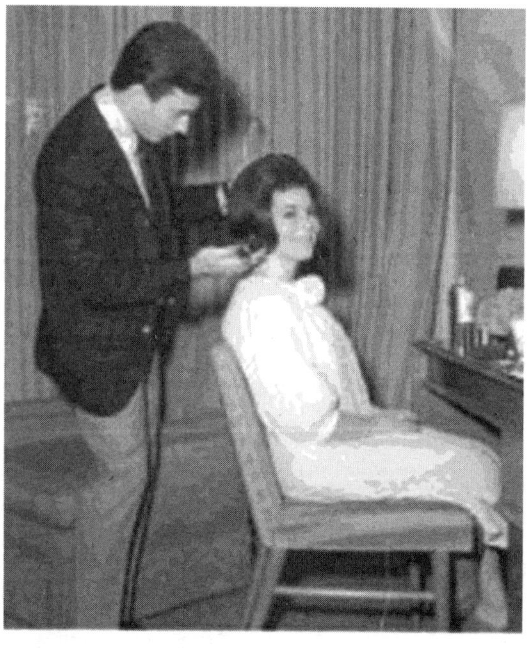

Yamanos was a Japanese beauty school, owned by Mike Yamano. It was where Norm was going to school and where I signed up the next day. It was mostly Japanese and Hispanic girls. Norm and I were the only two straight guys, and it was great fun. I also found that it came very easily to me, learning how to style hair. It was like playing the trumpet or dancing. I could be the star. (The Japanese would end up being a very big part of my life.)

At night, to make extra money, I parked cars for Frascati's Gourmet in Beverly Hills. I liked being around rich people and their cars. There's nothing like the smell of the wealthy. I love cars. I love anything flashy. I still remember some of the cars I parked. A 1963 Eldorado convertible was the hot car at the time. It still smelled of the beautiful blonde owner's perfume. It took me five minutes to get my nose off the seat.

Guys would pull up in 1963 Corvettes. I remember Charles Goulet, a fashion designer, pulled up in his 1950 Jaguar with two Afghan dogs in the back. He said to me as he was getting out, "Don't let the dogs out," and he started to go inside. The dogs immediately ran away. Then he said, very calmly, very fashionably, "Go get the dogs." Afghans are probably as fast as greyhounds. I said "no," but they returned a few minutes later.

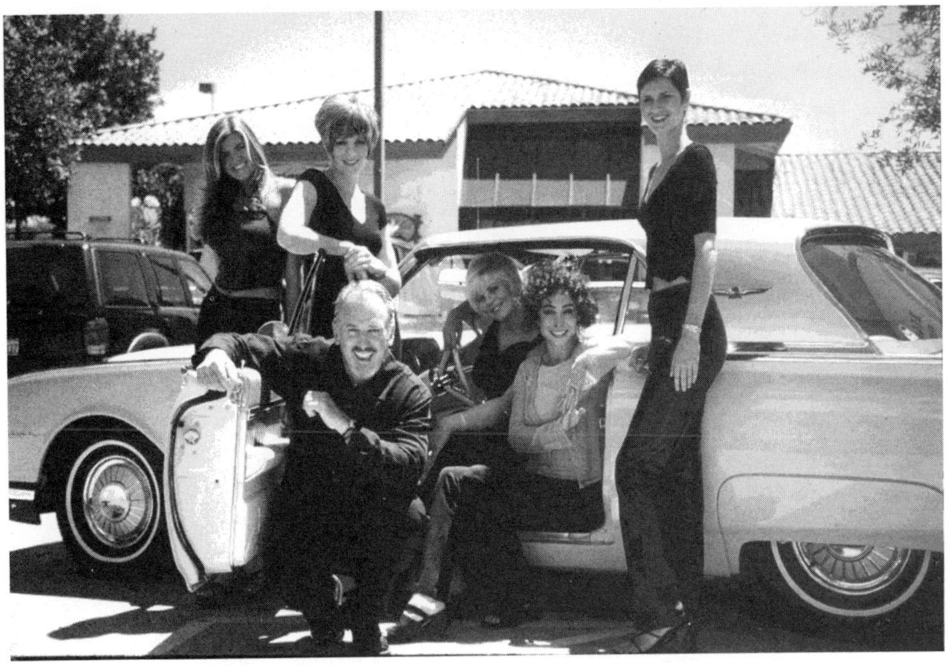

Me, years later. Old car, young girls. Love those cars.

I eventually got fired when I drove a Rolls Royce into a pole. I used to eat fried chicken and when I got behind the wheel of that Rolls, my hands slipped, and into the pole I went.

I also worked at May Company selling luggage. Got fired from there, too, for screwing a girl in the worker's lounge. (Those days were fun.)

But the one constant through it all, from way back in high school, was the lifestyle. The richness of it. I knew I had to live that way, which meant I had to be really good at beauty school. Just like when I was in junior high and high school, I had to be the best, or at least one of the best. At Yamanos, I definitely became the fastest, and made the most money. With that also came this horrendous 18-year-old ego.

In beauty schools, people come to get their hair done for very little money. With that, however, comes the possibility that you might end up with fried hair, blue hair, no hair. Unless people were lucky enough to get… Allen Goldstein. I was good. I got busier and busier, with Yamanos demanding more and more. I refused to work on older clients (no blue hairs for me) and when they forced me, I'd throw my little case of rollers at the wall. I was the star hairdressing student, throwing a tantrum.

I started doing house calls. I remember going to this one woman's house; she was old, at least 35, with two kids (remember: I was 18). I had this heavy, molasses-like stuff called wave-set. I was too lazy to put it into a smaller jar, so I tried to take the whole thing with me. When I took the lid off it spilled all over her. It was thick and gooey. It looked like snot. It smelled just as bad.

In those days, women teased their hair. Some women never washed their hair. (It was a very strange time. Very twilight zone.) Instead, they'd go to what was then called the beauty parlor, or the beauty school. One day I had this friend, not Norm, who was perming this woman's hair. He put the rollers in and ran the solution, and then went to lunch. Completely forgot about her. When he finally remembered and took the rollers out, her hair snapped off in the shampoo bowl. She screamed. That guy ran like one of those Afghans.

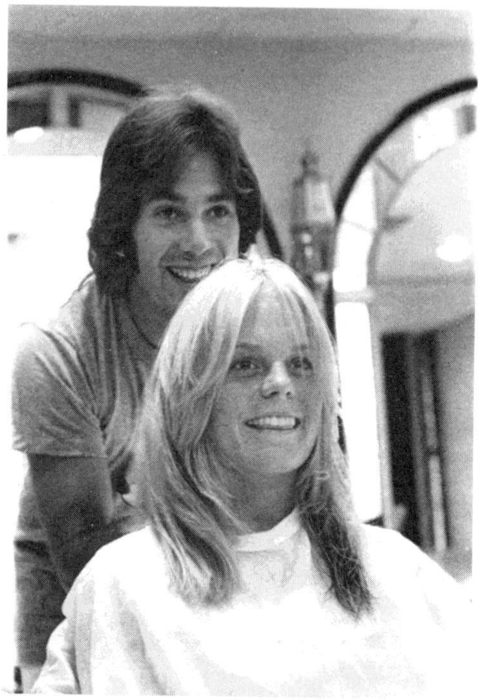

Me in the 1970s, behind the chair at Jon Peters.

After that, I immediately started cutting hair. It was Los Angeles, mid-1960s, and fashion was starting to show itself in Hollywood, on the Sunset Strip, everywhere. The beehive was famous, and I had one model at school whose hair was dyed jet black. I teased the hell out of her hair and made a beehive that was jet black and three feet tall. I put the top down in my car and drove down Sunset Boulevard on a Saturday night.

We sprayed hair with lacquer in those days. Pure lacquer. Today we use it to make wood shiny. I hated it.

The year flew by. It was easy and fun, and I started charging clients for getting their hair done by the world-famous now-19-year-old $2 extra or I wouldn't do them. I must have done something good though, because one of the clients I have now in the 21st century was someone whose hair I started doing in beauty school.

I was seriously dating a girl named Fran. I was also fooling around (no sex) with twenty other girls trying to get some action, not that I knew what action was. But it was OK because I wasn't serious with any of them.

Fran lived in a boarding house for girls in Hollywood called Hamburger House. I met her at a nightclub, and I wanted to impress her with my new Triumph Spitfire. She had a cute little bubble haircut and wore Empire dresses. She wanted to get married, but I wasn't sure. Maybe I wasn't sure I wanted to marry her. I always thought a relationship was based on fighting. That's what my parents had always done; that's what Fran and I started doing. And I didn't really like fighting, but I didn't know any better. It always seemed too counterproductive. So Fran wanted to be a married woman, and I was the guy she was dating. Still. I didn't know.

Something was lurking, though, that changed my mind. Vietnam. The rule was this: If you got married, you didn't have to go to Vietnam. So I got married. It was 1965. I thought, maybe, I loved her, too.

Flamenco

I graduated from Yamanos and my ego and I went to see a guy named Neal Sloane. In those days, he was one of the hottest hairdressers and salon owners around. There was also Gene Shacove, Carrie White, Richard Ocala, but not yet Vidal Sassoon. Neal hired me on the spot. I started immediately at his salon in Beverly Hills. Then I had a chance to go to a place called Flamenco, and it was my kind of place. Great looking women with lots of money driving incredible cars.

I had no clients, of course. But there was a girl who worked at the salon who was getting married, so she decided that she'd give me her clientele. I slept with her and then she decided she wasn't going to leave the salon after all (I was that good?) but that I could do her clients while she was on her honeymoon. I changed all of their hair while she was gone and ended up keeping them all.

I was the new guy, the young guy, and a lot of the women brought their daughters to me. I started doing a lot of models as well as hot young girls. There were a lot of extra bonuses, too, like if I was at the salon late, I could do a model's hair and then she could do me. The salon actually saved me money because I didn't have to pay for a hotel. Of course, the big dilemma was… do I still charge them? It didn't really feel like cheating because I barely knew who they were and it was part of the game, part of the time. I can honestly say that I lived during the time of the sexual revolution.

Fran, naturally, didn't like what I did for a living. Neither did her family. I was always the creative, artsy, wild one. She was attracted to that, but her family was pulling her in the opposite direction. Her mother had died when she was 16, and her older sister, Jan, ruled the roost. Uncle Alvin was the godfather of the family, and he announced I wasn't good enough for Fran. I was doomed.

I focused on building my clientele and being a great hairdresser. When the salon was sold to a guy named Peter Viser, my career took off. Peter was the first hairdresser I'd ever met who didn't tease hair. He did these great debutante women who arrived in Rolls Royces and limousines. I decided to become Peter Viser. I became the ultimate copycat. I could look at something he had done and do it as well. In those days, there was no training and no assisting. Peter had his own room, secluded from everyone. When he wasn't around I'd do his clients, but he didn't seem to mind. In fact, we became very good friends.

I stopped teasing hair and lost my entire clientele. But I was ready to move on. I liked the softness of what Peter was doing. The back brushing, the glamour, the make-over from long hair suddenly cut short, short getting bangs, blondes becoming redheads. Clairol was huge at that time, and red hair was the rage. It was very brash, like me.

I learned as much as I could from Peter and when I couldn't learn any more, I had to move on. That's when my father, who had always supported my decision to become a hairdresser, came to see me. He managed this apartment complex in Encino, and he had met this hot young guy who was opening a salon in Encino. My father told him about me,

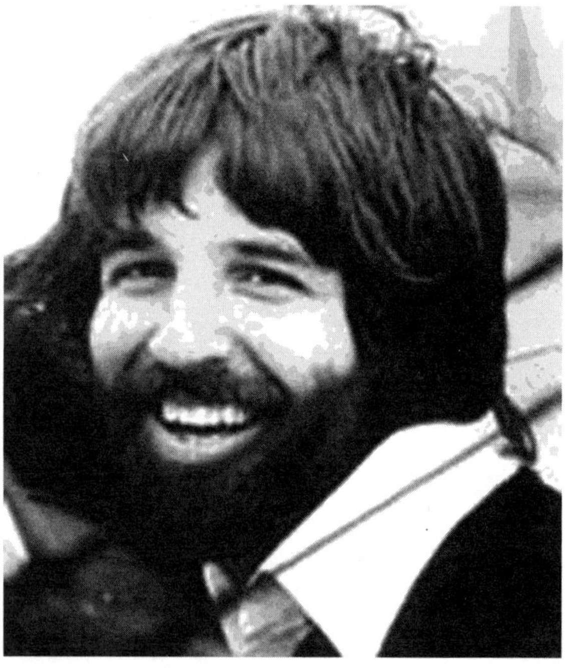

Jon Peters.

and they arranged a meeting at a night club on Sunset called Gazzari's. The guy drove up in a 1963 Corvette convertible with wide tires, lowered, with big black side pipes. He had this wild, dark hair and he climbed up and out of the car to introduce himself.

"Jon Peters," he said as he held out his hand.

"Al- Allen," I said. It was like meeting a rock star.

It seemed that Jon was opening a salon with another hairdresser named Paul Canter. Paul was the nice Jewish boy to Jon's aggressive Italian. He also had a lot of celebrity clients. I wanted to work with that type of mentor. So I met with the two of them, Paul and Jon, in their new 4,400-square-foot space, and they took me in. They were like father figures: Jon, the strong father; Paul, the good father. I was the hungry, eager-to-learn son.

Everything Jon taught me, I still use today. He developed this free way of cutting hair using tapering scissors. He was inspiring. He made me good at cutting hair, at reading hair. I picked up everything, including his defiant, creative personality, which I totally connected with. We were arrogant, drunk on power. Hairdressers really were rock stars back then. We didn't do anybody's hair that we didn't want to do.

Actually, forget rock stars. We were gods. Or we thought we were.

So there I was, married, 23, working for the hottest hairdresser in town, who also had one of the worst tempers I'd ever seen. I remember this pizza delivery guy who pissed Jon off, and Jon beat the shit out of him out on the sidewalk. That same pizza delivery guy came back one day and left a meat clever stuck in the middle of the front desk. And I thought that was great.

Fran liked Jon. She knew him from somewhere else, and as much as I admired him, there were moments when he really pissed me off. Little things would set him off. I scuffed my boots on the salon floor one day and he screamed at me in front of the staff. When he was done, I got in his face and very calmly said:

"If you ever do that again, I'll quit."

Tough talk from a tough kid.

Then he'd take me to car races and we'd have a blast. He was married to Lesley Ann Warren at the time, and we were at the house one morning. Some kid had parked his motorcycle on their front yard, and Jon was not happy. The kid thought he was really tough and so he hit Jon. I watched Jon wipe the blood from his mouth. Then he smiled.

"And now I'm going to kill you," he said and he beat the kid to a pulp. The kid ended up suing for assault, but Jon got off because he knew I would back him up (I did). I'd always do that for a friend. Besides, the kid was a real punk.

I wasn't a fighter, never really was. But I developed a black belt mouth.

Jon was doing celebrity clients like Jill St. John, Barbara Eden. She was actually a big thing for Jon until he got Lesley, and then *she* was the big thing. This was my first introduction to movie star clients.

It was 1973. I decided I was going to open my own salon, my first, in Woodland Hills. Paul got wind of it, and he and Jon decided that it was OK as long as they were my partners. We were going to call it Jon Peters Salon, Allen Goldstein, owner.

"Doesn't work," Jon said.

"Not at all," said Paul.

"I agree," I said. I decided then and there to start going by my first and middle name, with an 's.' Allen Goldstein became Allen Edwards. Owner.

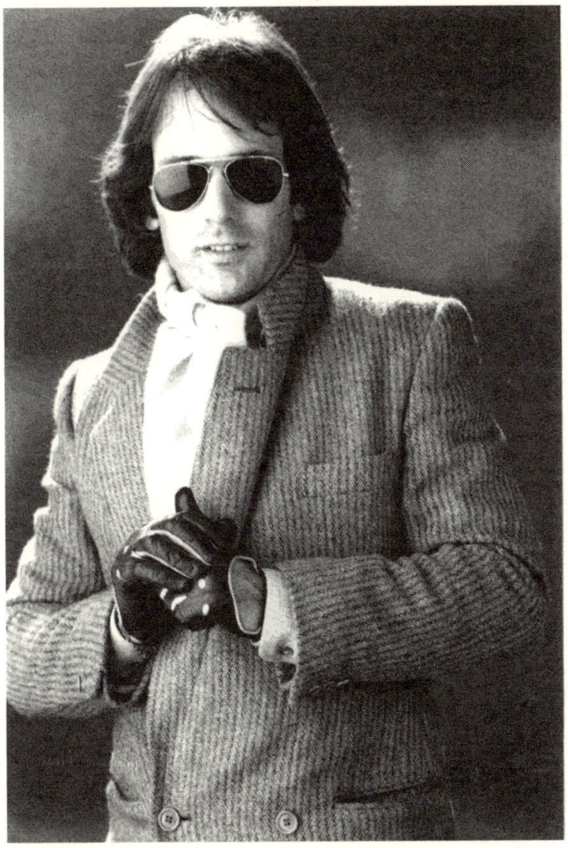

Me, in the '70s. Yeah. You're so vain.

Forget rock stars. We were gods.

three

Opportunity Knocks. I Answer.

The Farrah Fawcett

So the salon opened and it was called Jon Peters Salon, Allen Edwards, owner. There was no way my name wasn't going to be on that building. No way Jon was going to be the only star. Grudgingly, I had to admit that yes, it had Jon's name, but at that time Jon *was* the name; I was just the up and comer, the one with the new name. That was fine with me.

My dad hated the idea that I'd changed my name, though he never really shared his feelings on that. He just pulled away from me and our relationship became very thin. I can see now how he felt. It was like I was denouncing him, spitting on our heritage. I didn't think of it like that at the time. It was just a practicality thing. But I hurt him when I became Allen Edwards.

So the salon opened in Woodland Hills, a somewhat upscale area in the western end of the San Fernando Valley. One Saturday, the salon was packed. I had a rule: No children. This short, stocky guy came in. He had a black mole with a hair growing out of it. He also had his kids with him, who started screaming. I had my assistant ask him to leave. He walked by me, and with his baby in the baby stroller, he slammed through my brand new glass door. I lost it. I went out after him, leaving a salon full of clients with their mouths hanging open.

"Fuck you," he screamed. "All hairdressers are gay."

I went to throw a punch and my eye caught a glimpse of the mole. Which grossed me out. Jon's cousin, Silvio, who also worked at the salon, pulled me back. The police were called. Silvio said it was Mole-man who threw the first punch. The police left. Jon and I were even.

Shortly thereafter, Jon and Paul bought Pagannos, which had been owned by Jon's uncle, Adolph Paganno, who became partners with all of us. It was another hip salon in Beverly Hills, on Rodeo and Brighton. They had 4,000 square feet, which was a huge undertaking; I had 1,500 square feet. Much more manageable. Right around this time, Jon was branching out. He started to get into the movie business.

I remember going to talk to Jon when he was married to Lesley, when we were designing the Woodland Hills salon. They were naked. Jon was going through another wild stage, this time nudism. He loved shocking me, and it wasn't so much that I was shocked. It was that it was difficult talking to Jon when he was naked next to his wife, who was lying there on the lounge with that rockin' body. She and I still joke about that period of time. And she still looks hot.

Then they divorced. Jon started doing Barbra Streisand's hair. That relationship is legendary. He was the only person I knew who could go to a big star like Barbra and tell her that her hair looked like crap, that she was doing it all wrong, that she needed to change her whole image. And she'd change it. For him.

Jon invited me to Barbra's house one day in Beverly Hills when the relationship was first starting. It was so exciting to meet her. Her house was amazing, completely art deco. I left something there, went back the next day, walked in and she was singing with Burt Bacharach.

When Jon started living with Barbra, they bought a ranch in Malibu. That's when she started changing her look. She got rid of the long nails, permed her hair. This was pre-*A Star Is Born.* They had a pet lion cub. It was wild. We'd all go out to dinner at a place on Pacific Coast Highway called the Paradise Cove. Needless to say, we didn't have to wait for a table.

But I digress.

Movies were pulling Jon's interest from the hair business, which was just fine with me. Doors were opening for both of us.

During this time of building out the salon and getting it running, Paul and Jon weren't getting along at all. There may have even been some punching. For once, I didn't get involved. Besides, I always had the mentality of go for it, no matter what. Hey, opportunity was knocking. I just answered.

It took a year for Paul to break.

"I want you to buy out Jon," Paul said to me one day.

"You want me to buy out Jon," I said, sort of as a question, more as a statement.

"Yes," he countered.

"You want me (pause) to buy out Jon," I said again.

Paul nodded.

"You want me to buy out Jon?" I asked, the reality sinking in. The enormity of the request, the incredible possibilities that would exist for me if I did. The salons would no longer be Jon Peters Salons, but Allen Edwards Salons. Even Jon Peters Salon, Allen Edwards, owner, would be different. I would still be the owner, but it would just be my name. I wouldn't have to shout about it. I could just be it. Be the salon.

I would be the owner, the star, the name.

"OK," I said. OK. OK? Holy shit! What the hell was I thinking?

Obviously, of the future. Because shortly after Paul asked, my ambition got the better of me and I did it. I bought all three salons: Woodland Hills, Encino and Beverly Hills. I was the new boss. (With a lot more headaches.) Paul, Adolph and I became partners. A year later, Paul and I bought out Adolph.

Beverly Hills, 90210

My first day in Beverly Hills, they hated me. There was this group of four or five lunatics, Jon's cronies, and I was the new step-dad. So in typical Allen fashion, I thought "Fuck 'em." They were very gay and always drunk. The drug of choice? Quaaludes. But they were all great hairdressers. They were just reluctant, and yeah, wanted to get me out. They didn't know me at all. And I didn't know them. Except I did.

They were the most disgusting, drugged-out kooks to ever dress hair, but they were my kooks and I had to deal with them. And what they didn't get was that Jon was the one who trained me. I was Jon, 2.0, the updated model. Part of me had his same attitude. I had learned not to take shit from anyone.

It was the 1970s. Lots of drugs, lots of sex. Lots of money. Walking into that store that first day, with Jon being gone, was a humbling and empowering experience. His name, if not his atmosphere, remained. Paul and I decided that it would be best to keep his name around at least for a little while.

So there I am, the new daddy. And it was a disaster. They plotted against me. I had the attitude, I was the tyrant and nobody was supposed to fuck with me. I laid down the law: You dress the way I want, you look the way I want, use the scissors the way I want, blow out the hair the way I want. You get the idea. And of course, not one of them did what I wanted. Well, that wasn't entirely true. There were a couple of more conservative hairdressers that were on my side. It was about half of the salon. They became my team right away. They were great. I was also putting my own assistants on the floor. But the others, the ones who considered themselves Jon's people, they plotted. And plotted. And plotted. For four months.

One day, they took me outside. I'm thinking "What the hell?" They're thinking "We're going to set this guy straight." They were going to lay down their law, or they were going to quit. I was supposed to be afraid.

I wasn't.

I fired them all.

After that, my salons became the busiest in California (I have no scientific proof to back that up). We still were using Jon's name, but suddenly my name began appearing. I was getting press mentions, and Jon was completely out of the salon. I started doing some celebrity hair, or at least peripheral celebrity hair. I did Jane Brolin's hair, whose husband was James Brolin (who eventually became husband to Barbra Streisand… talk about the small world syndrome).

The Beverly Hills salon was busy, but completely different than being in Woodland Hills. Woodland Hills was delicate. Beverly Hills wasn't. One day this girl tipped me with a little vial of white powder. Being a nice Jewish Valley boy, I didn't know what it was. I dropped it by accident and it hit the ground and rolled out the door. There was this hush of silence.

"What is that?" I asked innocently. Honest.

Nobody said anything. But I got it, finally. I let it go. Somebody somewhere was very happy that day. And I was kind of pissed off I didn't just get a twenty.

In Beverly Hills, you had to wait at least half an hour to get shampooed. Raquel Welch would go crazy waiting, screaming in the back, but by the time she got to my chair, she was fine.

Still, Jon haunted the place. He was my mentor; he was the best. Even his bad parts seeped into me, and I used them to become better at what I was doing.

Jane Brolin was friendly with a minor celebrity who was starting to gain some notoriety largely because she was married to the Six-Million Dollar Man. Her name was Farrah Fawcett-Majors. One day this pretty, athletic blonde walked into the salon with her hair all one length and wanting something different. This was pre-*Charlie's Angels* and during Wella-Balsam commercials. Before she developed her huge bullshit attitude. We hit it off and I started cutting her hair.

The big change was multiple layers and cutting the front shorter to create what would quickly become the "Farrah" look. It took on a life of its own. Everyone wanted the "Farrah" cut. That's when I invented a method called blow-curl. It was a way of setting the hair with a blow dryer and clips.

I started traveling with her during the commercials. I never got close to her though. One of her good friends was Jose Eber, but he wasn't doing her hair at the time. I was. (Let's get that straight right now.) But whatever relationship we had went from really good to total shit. Maybe it started to end when she went on the *Merv Griffin Show* and he asked about her hair. She said she did it herself. I'm still picking up the pieces of the television set I threw against the wall. And the funny thing was, she had an appointment the next day. I was infuriated.

Next day. She walked in. Sat down in my chair. I fumed.

"I saw you on Merv," I said finally. It went downhill from there.

Her hair was becoming more famous than her. And all I could think was, in the world of celebrity, if you say you do your own hair, maybe you should do your own hair. I threw her out of the salon.

When I did Marcia Clark's hair, much later, in the mid 1990s, when O.J. Simpson was on trial for the murder of his ex-wife, Farrah's lawyer sent me a letter telling me not to say I did Farrah's hair. I sent a picture of the two of us back to her lawyer with a nice little note that said, "I hope Farrah feels better. Apparently she's having a memory problem."

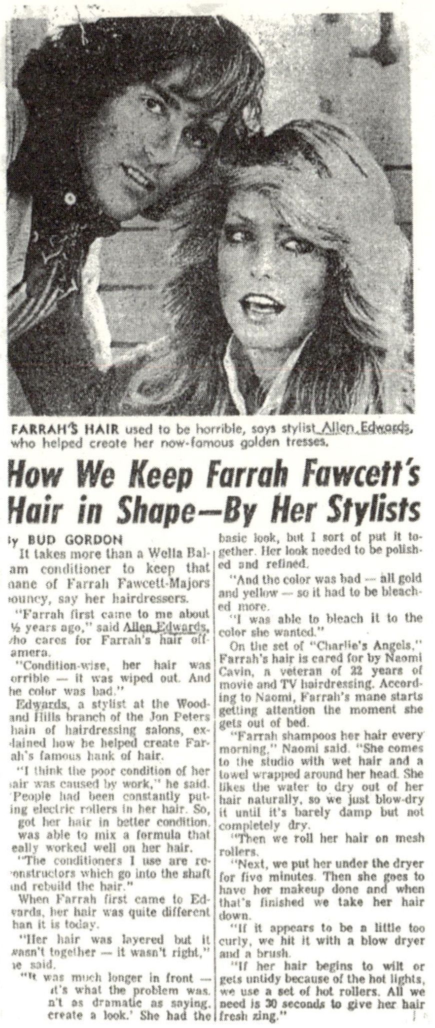

FARRAH'S HAIR used to be horrible, says stylist Allen Edwards, who helped create her now-famous golden tresses.

How We Keep Farrah Fawcett's Hair in Shape—By Her Stylists

ɜy BUD GORDON

It takes more than a Wella Balam conditioner to keep that nane of Farrah Fawcett-Majors ɔouncy, say her hairdressers.

"Farrah first came to me about ½ years ago," said Allen Edwards, who cares for Farrah's hair offamera.

"Condition-wise, her hair was orrible — it was wiped out. And he color was bad."

Edwards, a stylist at the Woodand Hills branch of the Jon Peters hain of hairdressing salons, exlained how he helped create Farah's famous hank of hair.

"I think the poor condition of her ıair was caused by work," he said. 'People had been constantly puting electric rollers in her hair. So, got her hair in better condition. was able to mix a formula that eally worked well on her hair.

"The conditioners I use are reonstructors which go into the shaft ınd rebuild the hair."

When Farrah first came to Edvards, her hair was quite different han it is today.

"Her hair was layered but it wasn't together — it wasn't right," ıe said.

"It was much longer in front — it's what the problem was. n't as dramatic as saying. create a look.' She had the basic look, but I sort of put it together. Her look needed to be polished and refined.

"And the color was bad — all gold and yellow — so it had to be bleached more.

"I was able to bleach it to the color she wanted."

On the set of "Charlie's Angels," Farrah's hair is cared for by Naomi Cavin, a veteran of 22 years of movie and TV hairdressing. According to Naomi, Farrah's mane starts getting attention the moment she gets out of bed.

"Farrah shampoos her hair every morning," Naomi said. "She comes to the studio with wet hair and a towel wrapped around her head. She likes the water to dry out of her hair naturally, so we just blow-dry it until it's barely damp but not completely dry.

"Then we roll her hair on mesh rollers.

"Next, we put her under the dryer for five minutes. Then she goes to have her makeup done and when that's finished we take her hair down.

"If it appears to be a little too curly, we hit it with a blow dryer and a brush.

"If her hair begins to wilt or gets untidy because of the hot lights, we use a set of hot rollers. All we need is 30 seconds to give her hair fresh zing."

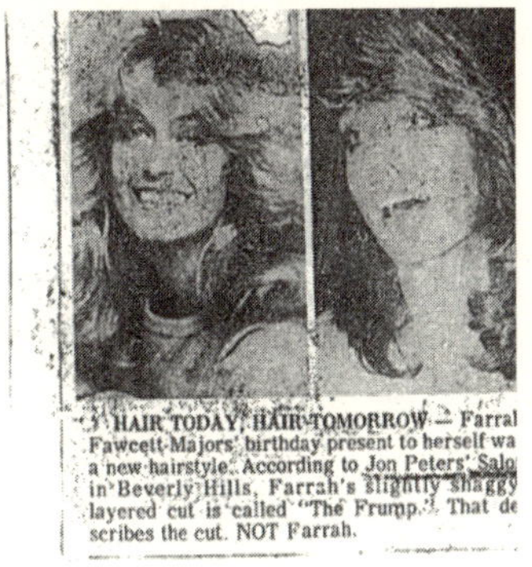

HAIR TODAY, HAIR TOMORROW — Farral Fawcett-Majors' birthday present to herself wa a new hairstyle. According to Jon Peters' Salo in Beverly Hills, Farrah's slightly shaggy layered cut is called "The Frump." That de scribes the cut. NOT Farrah.

Farrah always tried to give credit to Jose Eber, which wasn't his fault. Even now, I won't say anything bad about him. He's a great competitor of mine. A talented guy. The biggest problem with some celebs is that they're afraid to give credit to other people. Especially in the '70s and '80s. People were so known for their hairstyles that they wanted to believe and they needed everyone to believe it was their creation.

Raquel Welch was the same way. When I cut her hair short, she took credit for it. But I had already called the *Los Angeles Times* to tell them. I was going to get the credit. Hairdressers are such an important part of making celebrities look good. They need to give credit to their hairdressers and makeup artists. Though I think today's celebs are better than yesterday's celebs, the problem is that today's hairdressers don't seem to put the effort out to get the press. What's up with that?

Even with all of the crap, Farrah was and remains a tremendous door opener for me. The *New York Times* listed it as one of the greatest haircuts of all time. *Allure* magazine in August 2006 wrote about it. It was in a summer 2007 issue of *Entertainment Weekly.* (Still!) I always wanted to be known for *what* I do, not *who* I do. That's what stays with me.

Growl is worse than the bark

Charlie's Angels started in 1975, which, coincidentally, was the same year I started doing a little something called *The Regis Show,* with Regis Philbin and Sarah Purcell. I'd strut out onto the stage, under the hot lights, in front a cheering audience, in a white suit and scarf. No one had ever seen a hairdresser on television before, and there was Allen, bigger than life. In a small box.

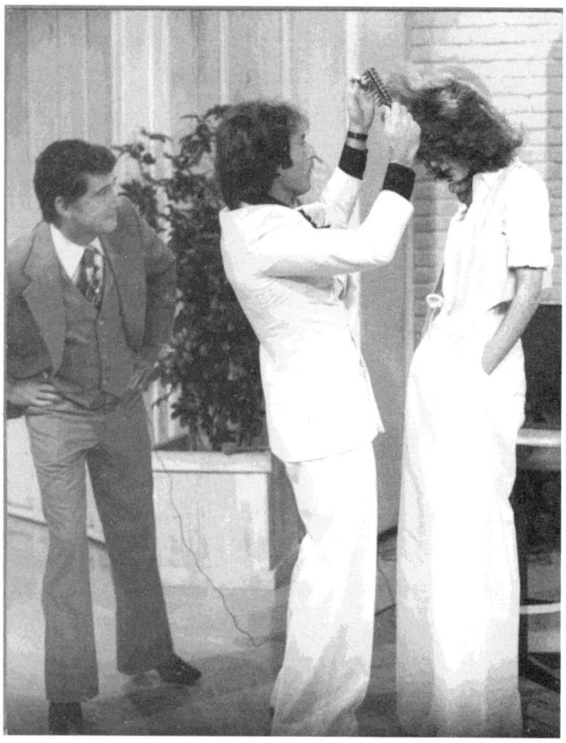

Me on the set of The Regis Show.

And what does Regis do on that first show? Announce me as the creator of the one, the only, the fabulous… Farrah Fawcett. Not the woman, of course. The hair. The salon got 500 phone calls that first day.

So there I was on TV, the stutterer. Scared shitless. But I never stuttered once. I did four models that first day, showed off new looks, new ideas. I showed off the Blow Curl where I blow-dried the hair, rolling it around a small brush, hitting it with heat. And I just knew then that television was going to change my life.

Television also gave me the power to introduce women all over the country to different looks and different haircuts. I had people writing me letters from all over. Farrah was followed by Sally Field, Anne Bancroft, Rene Russo, Suzanne Somers, Geena Davis and many more, and they were all followed by the press. Suddenly, Allen Goldstein from Canoga Park by way of Hollywood by way of Chicago, was hot stuff. I got a PR firm, I became personal friends with Regis, started doing Regis' wife's hair, and a year to the day after I bought out Jon Peters, I took his name off of the salons and put mine up.

Allen Edwards Salon.

Finally.

The Salon

I was married. I was having one affair after another, mostly with married women because they already had husbands. It was free; it was casual; it was the time. It was almost not cheating because it was the 1970s, a crazy time when the women wanted it just as bad as the men. (I hear they still do, though I'm now happily married, and way too tired.)

Then I met Lisa, the woman who would eventually become my second wife, the love of my life, a leggy brunette with a cute bob, dressed in coveralls, and my heart skipped a beat. No, two. Hell, maybe a bunch. She was married, too, but she was off limits at that time. Go figure. I just grew some morals. Right there, in an Allen Edwards Salon.

I was a hairdresser's hairdresser and I loved that. I trained hundreds of stylists to do great hair and then go out on the floor. I taught classes at least twice a week, and I started to make some real money. Which I needed because I had toys to buy… Porsches, Jags,

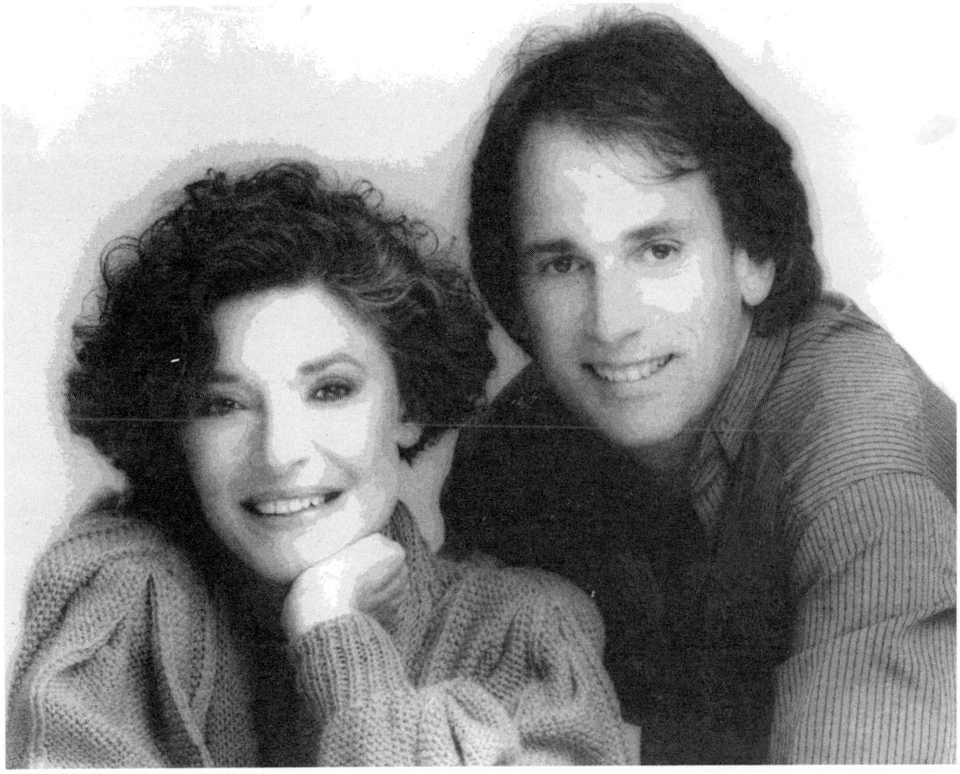

Me, with the late, great Anne Bancroft. She was a client for twenty years.

boats and bikes. Because I was short, it was always about how much horsepower was under the hood. (My first bike was so small it looked like I was riding a dog.)

Believe it or not, I was also trying to be a better husband and father. I had a daughter then, Amy, who was the love of my life. And then my dad died. I was devastated. But still, I lived to do hair. (I still do.) I went to every show, I took advantage of every opportunity to be in the spotlight. I was a star with shears. What Vidal Sassoon had accomplished in the 1960s, with famous clients like Mia Farrow and Twiggy, I was doing in the '70s, creating famous looks. The Farrah. The Scrunch, the Raquel Welch short haircut, the Donna Mills bob. These weren't makeovers; they were new looks created from new ideas.

One of my best experiences ended up being with Raquel Welch, creating her hair for the cover of French *Vogue*. The photographer was Scavullo, one of the most famous photographers in the world. Then she asked me to do her hair for the Emmy Awards. I went to her house, put electric rollers in her hair. One of the rollers got stuck, knotted in her hair.

"What's a matter, darlin'?" she drawled.

"Nothing. Nothing." Shit. Shit. Finally, I got it out. She looked great.

Doing Donna Mills' hair was another great experience. She was one of my favorite celebrity clients and became a good friend. I met her at a function. She was there with Beverly Sassoon, but we hit it off. Donna was one of the most famous women on television at the time as the star of *Knots Landing*, and she was always there for me.

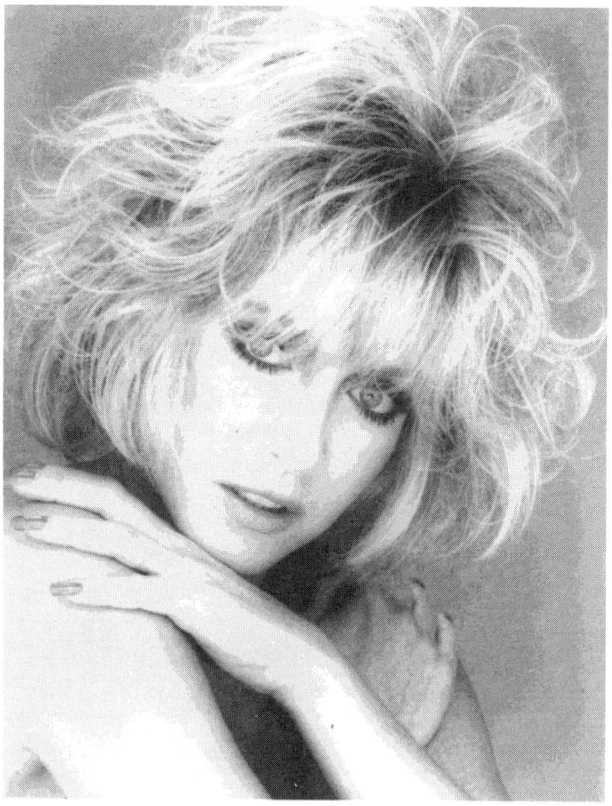

My friend and client, Donna Mills.

We had a shoot for *Redbook* one day, to show her new haircut. The photographer was a very flamboyant guy from New York. Donna liked to be a lit a certain way. She told me to go tell him that his lighting was wrong.

"You've got to be kidding," I said.

"Yes, go tell him," she said.

Being totally dominated by her, I went over to the guy and whispered in his ear, "Donna hates your lighting."

He threw a tantrum and Donna walked out.

That afternoon, *Eye on LA* did a whole show on me. She showed up and was her usual fabulous self. I finally got to show her new look, the scrunched bob. She opened many doors for me and changed the way women did their hair. Women all over started scrunching.

I also did the cover of *Time* magazine with Diane Keaton when she did *Annie Hall*, right when the movie came out. It was before she won all those awards, including the Oscar®. Later I'd go do her hair at Warren Beatty's house, and I'd walk into the living room and there would be Beatty and Nicholson, as in Jack. It was wild.

There are a lot of creative hairdressers. Who can say who's the best? It's like acting. It's an art, a craft that you learn. Some people just go different directions with it. I think people have to really learn what they do well, educate themselves and go as far as they can with it. Whether it's designing a house or building a motorcycle. Go for it. Go as far as you can. There's no such word as failure. (It's just not an option.)

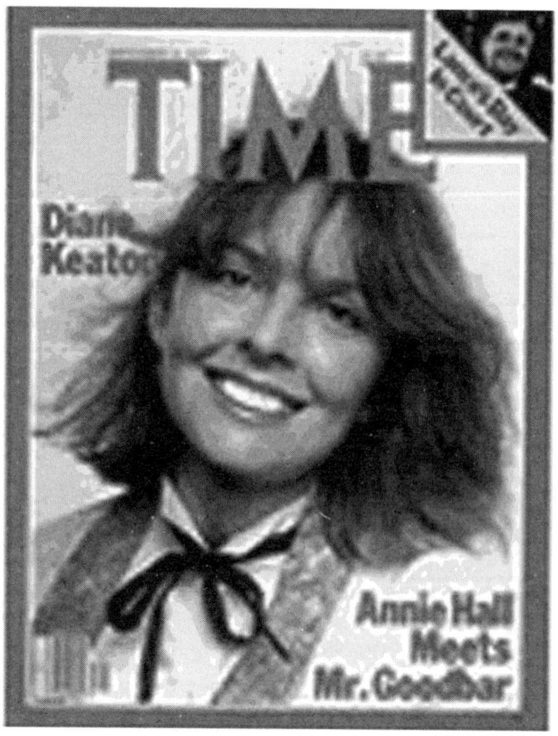

Diane Keaton on the cover of Time.

I used to tell my partner to tell me what I did bad because I already knew what I was doing good. That's the only way I could improve, by knowing the bad. Sometimes my ego got in the way and I disagreed, but it's important to know what you can improve on. Constructive criticism will only help you grow and get better. Put the big ego in the closet.

Life really isn't a contest. There are no winners or losers, unless it's something you enter. I never really liked going into competitions. I don't like to lose. I like to do what I do best, going on TV, going on stage. In a contest, I'm setting myself up for the potential to lose, and I'm not interested in that.

I was always hungry to be on stage. I was obsessed with being in the spotlight. I was constantly hounding my PR people to get me out there. And if they couldn't do it, they got fired.

I came from the era of creating a new haircut, not just a new look, and in Allen Edwards Salons, it was always about showing the new haircut. Television pushed me to come up with new concepts, which was incredibly hard. Then I started coming up with concepts: Hair to go to bed in; Mother's Day hair. Hairdos created with wet hair. I even did a show once about women who look like their dogs. In a good way.

Oh, the possibilities.

A lot of hairdressers get on TV, get their 15 minutes. But for me, once my time on TV was over, I had to move on to the next thing, the next sensation. It was never enough. Even later, when my second wife opened an exercise studio, I had to put my name on it: Allen Edwards Body Heat. I wanted the recognition. And I could get my name out there while also promoting the salons, with the exercise studio. But that was later.

Then …

"OK. That's over. What's next?"

That's why my salons have always had such longevity. It always feels like the beginning to me.

Then I started looking at fashion. Western wear hair? Yee-haw. Yeah, right. Who was I kidding? I was working five to six days a week, and constantly reinventing something I could take on TV. I craved the spotlight, and I couldn't get enough of it. I always worked to make the moment special for the audience.

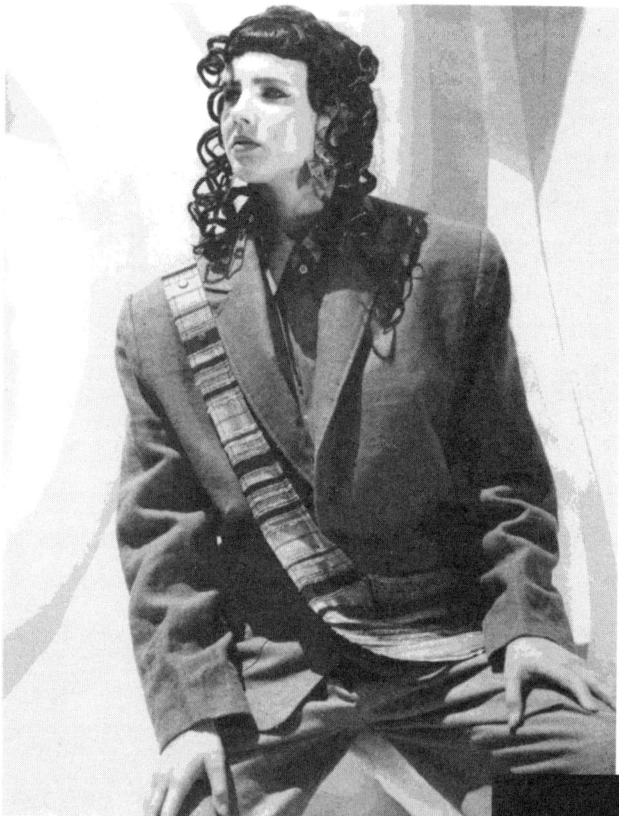

Oh, the possibilities.

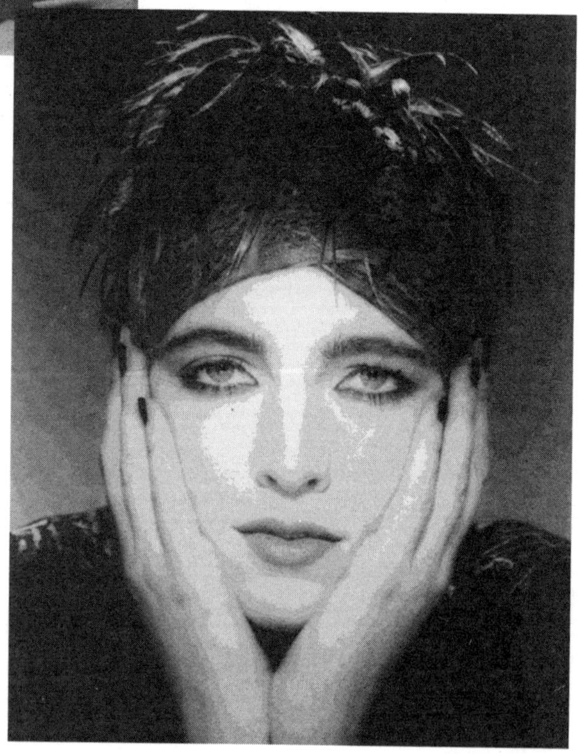

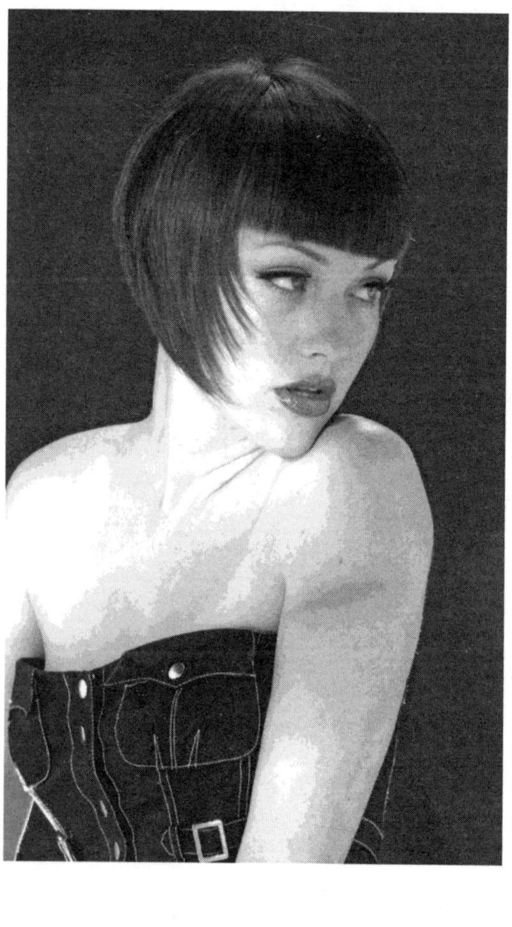

I remember doing Regis' show when Sarah Purcell was the co-host, when Mary Hart was the co-host, when Kathie Lee Gifford was the co-host. I did all of their hair.

I also did Cristina Ferrare's hair when she was with Steve Edwards. Then she left me and went to Christof, who would do her hair at 5 AM. What made Christof famous was when he did President Clinton's hair on the tarmac at LAX. He was always a very personal, not in-your-face hairdresser.

I was doing it all, doing all of the talk show hosts' hair. I got so confident I even took the producer of the *Regis Show* out to dinner and wanted to know how I could get my own talk show. That was good for a laugh. And a rude awakening. People don't look at hairdressers as talk show people.

"This isn't what you do. It's not what you're known for," he said. "If Regis quit, we'd go to someone who had talk show experience."

It was a great lunch.

But I tried. If you don't try, you can't succeed.

I had watched Regis go through co-host after co-host. One was the aforementioned Mary Hart, and they asked me to do her hair. They wanted a famous photographer, Michael Childers, to do a photo shoot. I convinced her to cut all of her hair off, and she did. She was very young and very hot. I got to be in the photo shoot as well, and *Eye on LA* filmed me cutting off all her hair. She was a great client throughout her career, right up until she married Burt Sugarman. He wanted her to be blonder, and I didn't believe she should be (she's really dark) because it would show her roots too much. But I did it. I made her blonder against my better judgment, and she was unhappy and wanted it fixed. Her secretary called me right before Christmas.

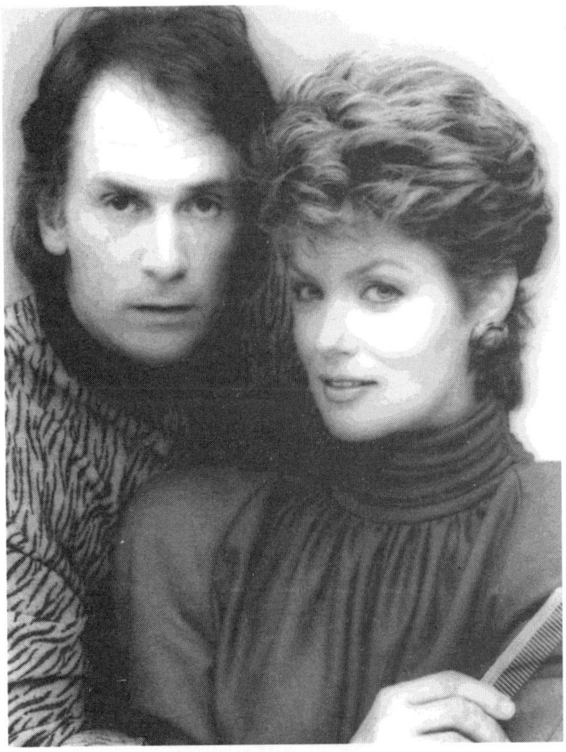

Mary Hart. It was good while it lasted.

"Either you do it Sunday, or you don't see her anymore," her secretary said.

"Well, then I don't see her," I said. I had a Christmas party planned for the Sunday in question. I went to the party, not to Mary's house, and that was that. Once you start talking to someone's assistant or secretary, you know you're in trouble.

Mary dumped me. But I wasn't bitter.

So right about this time, I was running the two Hills: Woodland and Beverly. And the salon in Encino, which was run by Paul, had a hairdresser named Geri Cusenza. She was a phenomenon. Incredibly talented. Incredibly ambitious. (Full disclosure: Geri was married to a man named John Sebastian and they started the hair care product line by the same name.) She was probably one of the best hairdressers I have ever known. She had also just created a little thing called The Crimping Iron.

Geri convinced Paul to let her train hairdressers as educators so that they could then educate other hairdressers about her iron and a protein treatment called 2 + 1. She also promised that she would never open a salon of her own. She was a liar.

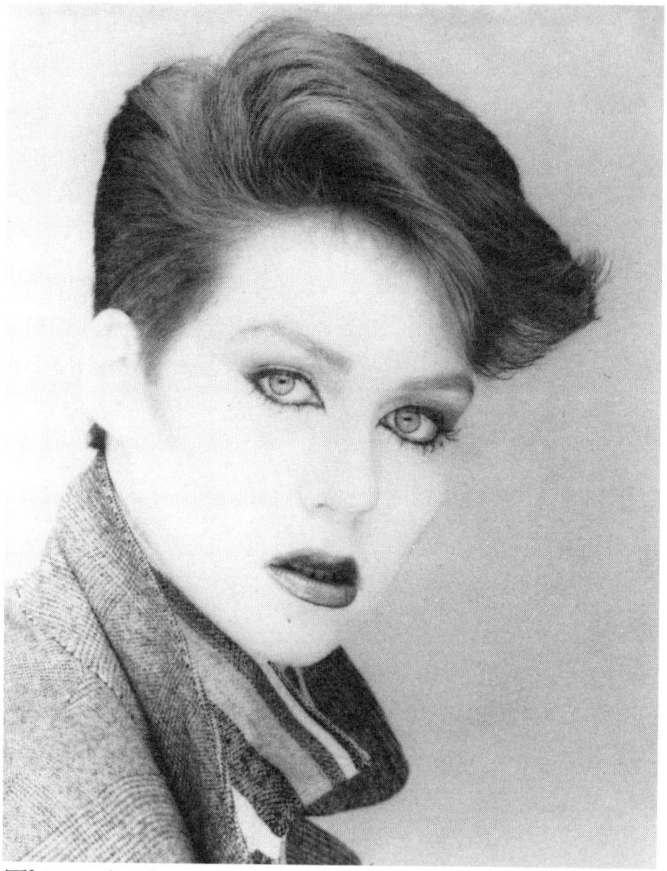

This isn't Geri, but it could be. This model, actually done in the 1980s, looks just like her. She was many things… including beautiful.

Two months later, I was cruising down Ventura Boulevard and I saw this amazing building, and I knew it had to be hers. I could tell from the design. (Don't ask me how. You have to know Geri to understand.) I asked the guy working there about the owners. Big surprise: Geri Cusenza and John Sebastian. I wanted to drive my big black Bronco through the front windows.

I went back to the salon and fired everyone she had been involved with. She took 27 of my people from Encino and five people from Woodland Hills and opened a salon called Cassandra. She got all my hairdressers plus Sebastian. I got empty salons.

Rule one of the hairdresser wars: Trust no one.

But who originally trained her hairdressers? Allen Edwards.

Rule two: Know who you are.

Because of my TV exposure and my PR, I built the salon back up within a year. Geri ended up closing Cassandra and a lot of the hairdressers came back to me.

Beverly Hills 911

I was always tormented by the little Allen sitting on my shoulder (yeah, even after I thought I killed him, he kept coming back), telling me that I wasn't going to make it. The salon on Rodeo was still the flagship, and Beverly Hills was still the place to go for shopping, fashion and beauty. I was about to find out just how "still the place" it was.

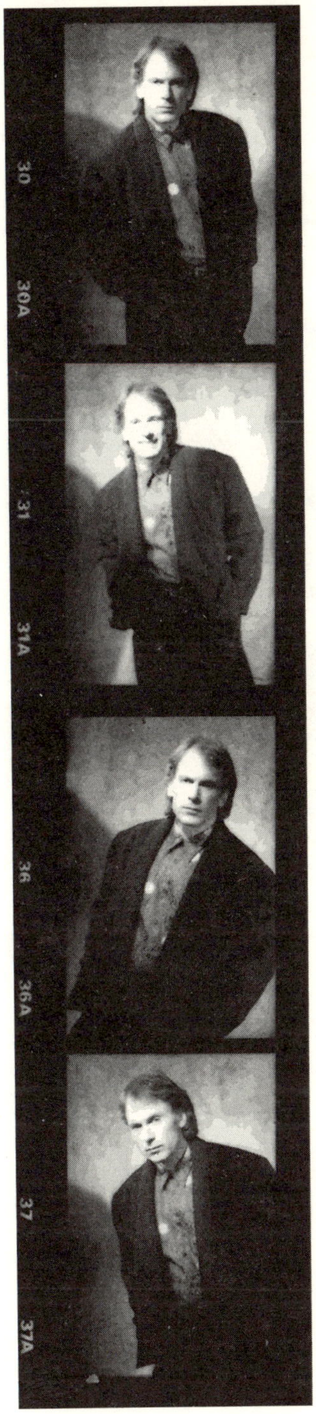

Know who you are.

"Your rent's going up a little bit," said my business manager.

"What's a little bit?" I asked.

"Well, we've been paying about $2,500 a month. But it's going up to $10,000."

"A month?" I asked. Shouted, actually.

He nodded.

"Rent is going up by $7,500 and you think that's a little bit?"

"I was trying to soften the blow," he said.

"Why?" I asked.

"Well, I figured that—"

"No. Why is it going up so much?"

"Well..."

Rodeo Drive had become famous. So now we had to pay for the privilege of such an address. Somehow I didn't feel all that privileged.

I happened to be friends with a woman named Gwen Jones who worked at the (now defunct) *Herald-Examiner*. She printed a story about how the rent had quadrupled. A guy named Wally Mark, who owned the building where my Beverly Hills salon lived, had major bucks and liked the idea of three hair salons in his building: first Shacove, then Sassoon, and now me. He offered me different space for less money. It was still in Beverly Hills. I jumped at the chance. I remodeled the new space and it became a fantastic salon.

Did I mention I was still in Beverly Hills?

Lesson: one part of life can be going really smooth while another part can be falling apart. Concentrate on the best part and the other will change. It's the glass half full, half empty thing.

Lesson, part 2: multiple businesses can help support each other.

I also continued to do what I do best. Hair. Teaching. Showing up on stage. It helped keep everything afloat. I knew I could always fall back on cutting hair. That gave me security, and security gave me strength.

The late 1970s

Along with the Farrah Fawcett and Beverly Hills and platform shoes came platform hair shows. Sebastian may have been one of the first professional hair care companies to spring up during the '70s, but it wasn't the last. Paul Mitchell, Nexxus, Aveda and KMS were also born during this decade, and with these manufacturers came artistic shows, created specifically to entice other hairdressers to reach for the stars.

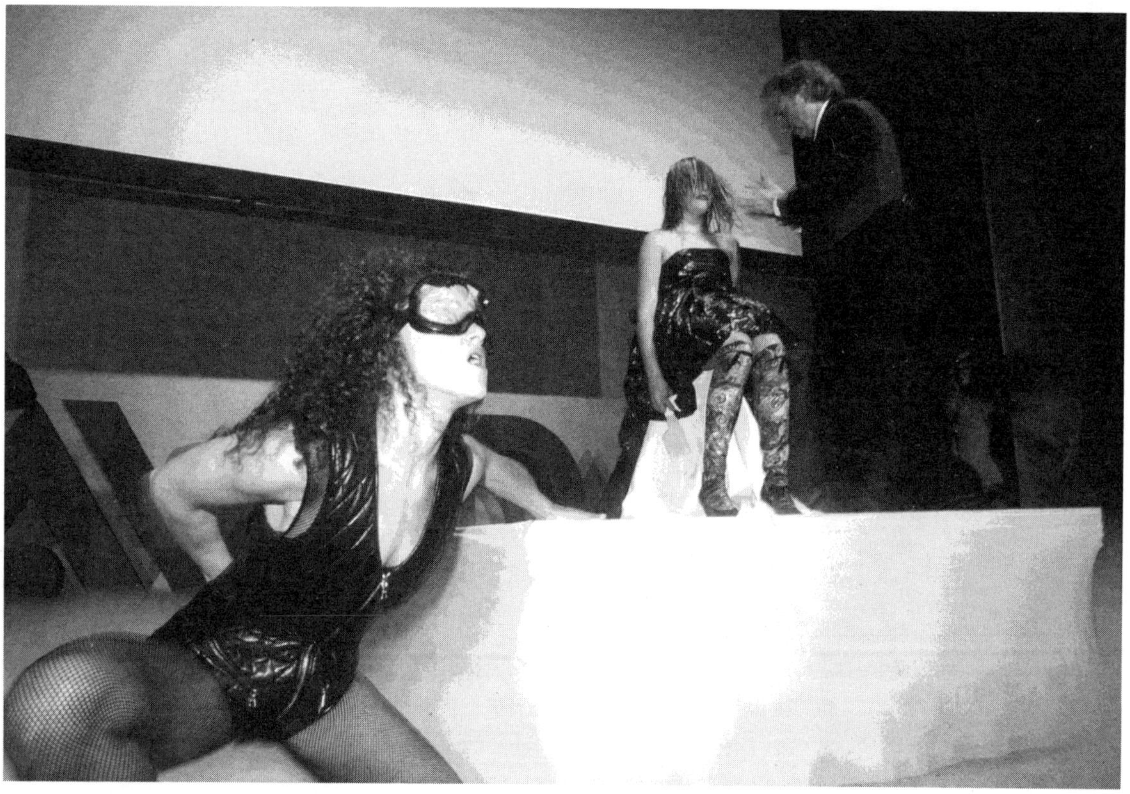

On stage.

Now remember. I loved the spotlight. Loved being on stage. Somebody at KMS had obviously seen me and decided that I would be a good person to front their stage shows, to represent them. His name was Mike Fazio. Should I take it? Damn right.

The first show was in front of 5,000 hairdressers. You'd think I'd stutter being in front of that many people at one time. (TV didn't count. I couldn't see the audience, so I could pretend they weren't there.)

It was called "Follow the Yellow Brick Road to Your Success." I was going to produce a show that was like a rock concert. There were dancers, dry ice. (My future wife, Lisa, was a dancer. I wanted her in the troupe. They hired her. Thank God she was good.) Smoke filled the stage and the audience was completely hushed. From the mist, I emerged. My act was cutting hair to music, using 7" scissors and a wild, high energy beat. I had learned how to cut hair very fast with very large scissors. I'd be out there alone, cutting. No words, nothing but music and hair flying everywhere.

"And now… ALLEN EDWARDS!"

That was my call to arms. I was standing backstage and before I came out, I was almost lethargic, gearing up. Then the music started pounding, my name was announced and there was this explosion of adrenaline.

Then came the teaching part, when 10 other hairdressers came out, cutting 25 models. It was like a rock and roll show, and I was finally where I should be.

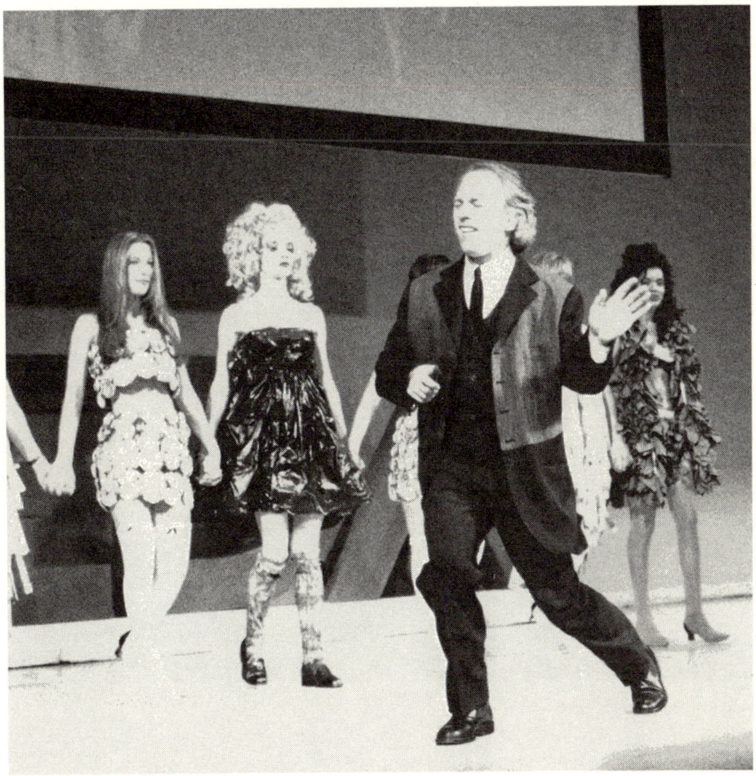

Still on stage for Aveda, dancing in front of 5000.

Hair was flying everywhere. We used music from *The Wiz* and Michael Jackson (he was still considered cool then… how the mighty have fallen), and I was weaving around the stage with a microphone. I talked for two hours. Teaching, explaining, encouraging, inspiring. I didn't want to lose the audience, not even for a second. I was hyper as hell. It was the first of many such shows.

I'd always end the show the same way: me cutting hair, with dancers swirling around me as the big finale. I wanted to have 5,000 people rush the stage when the last note sounded. I wanted them to come for a rock and roll fantasy, done with hair, and leave being proud of their chosen profession.

The thing I was most proud of? My team. We always got a standing ovation. Oh, and no stuttering.

At that time, we were making $5,000 a show.

Then I was hired to do a show in Boston. I put together something entirely different using music from Queen (remember, this was the 1970s). My hairdressers and I took the stage to the driving beat of "We Will Rock You." Then this high energy, classical music started to play. The energy was astounding. We could have powered the whole city that night from the stage.

I had this need to excite thousands of people at one time. I even started using some comedy bits, hair experiences and anecdotes, humorous tales woven throughout the presentation. Anything to further endear me to my audience. My team thought I was becoming too funny. I disagreed. The audience laughed, they cheered, and they learned.

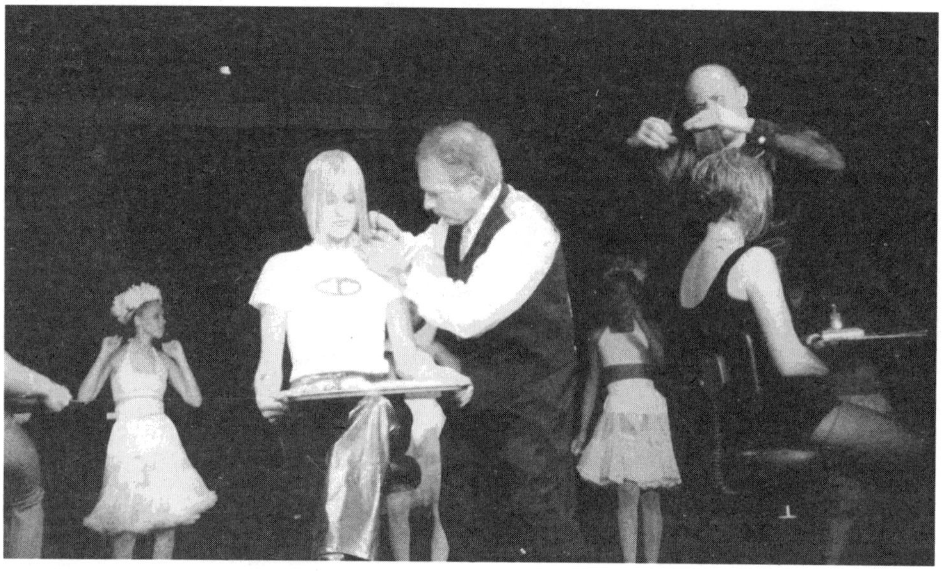

Boston.

In the Boston audience was a man named Mel Joseph, who worked for Clairol. He'd never seen anything like what was onstage in front of him. He went to my next show, in Atlantic City, just to see if it was a fluke. It wasn't. He hired me on the spot to represent Jazzing (a semi-permanent hair color designed to compete with Sebastian's Cellophanes) in ten shows. My answer: "Fuck yes!"

Coincidentally, right around this time, American Salon put up two names for hairdresser of the year: Geri Cusenza and Allen Edwards. Guess which guy won?

I became the highest paid platform artist in the country. I flew first class, had limousines transfer me around. My competition was always Sebastian. Their shows were ridiculously expensive to produce. Hundreds of thousands of dollars. I could do a show for a fraction of that. I did the planning, the hiring, the editing. I was the energy source—just plug me in—and I loved every minute of it. I still got standing ovations. A standing ovation is a standing ovation. And there's nothing like it.

I think the audience loved our shows because they could relate to me, because I was talking from the heart about how to be a great hairdresser, what "the look" is about. It was about tapping into the passion of doing hair. I still feel the same way.

What makes a great hair show is stimulating the people watching you. What made my shows different was that I turned these people on to the energy of hair.

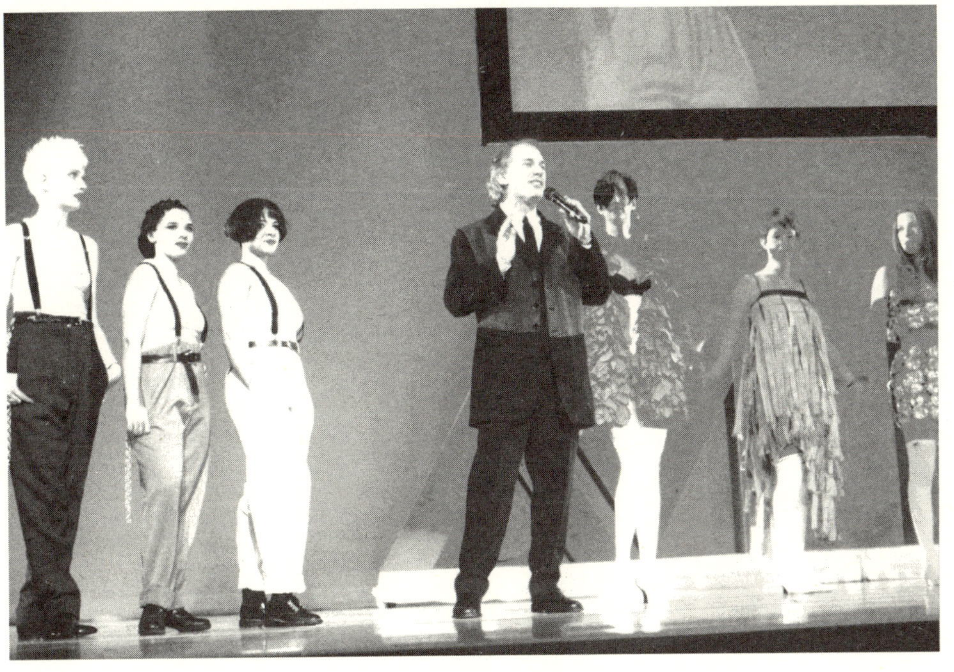

Yes. Still on stage.

I made $10,000 per show with Clairol. It was wild, a total party extravaganza every time there was a show.

To some of the major companies, I was the wild card, the rock star. They never knew what I was going to say and do, and that scared people. I liked that.

I now had two children, Amy and my son Jason. And I was wilder than ever.

I could only imagine what was next.

It was wild, a total party extravaganza.

four

I was king. Sort of.

So I was a success. I owned salons, which now sported only my name. I was on stage; I was in the public eye. I was rockin'. I had learned from Jon the power of celebrity. I had learned to take advantage of people, in a good way. Not to exploit them, but to utilize them to help my career. I knew that when it came to hair, people wanted to see beauty, femininity. They wanted to see sexy. Look at the "Farrah Fawcett," the "Donna Mills," the "Raquel Welch." All sexy. All designed by me. No ego here. (I was the king.)

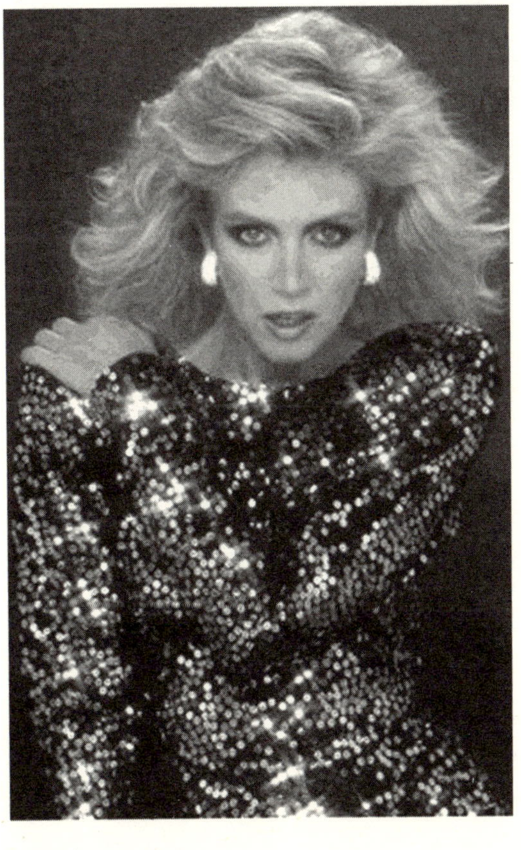

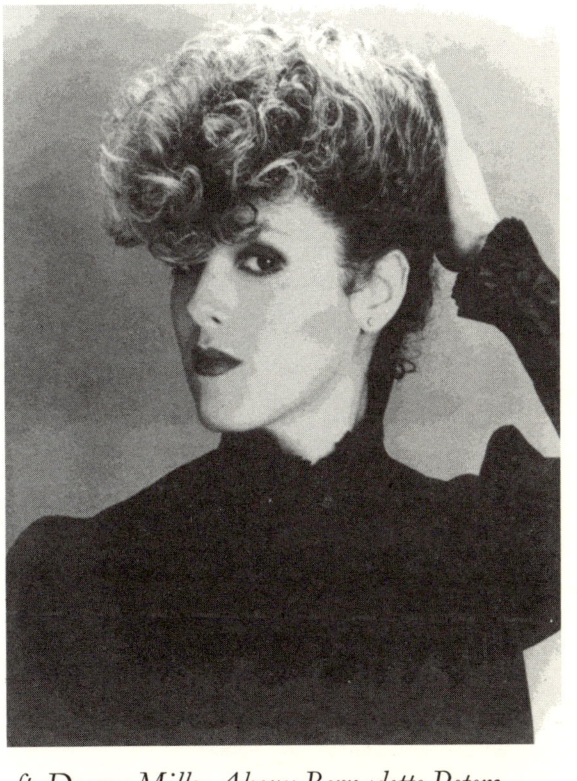

Left: Donna Mills. Above: Bernadette Peters.

I got a publicist and started pushing the public relations aspect of my business. It made me a known commodity, which made my salons busy, which made the hairdressers busy, which made me happy. And I loved the idea that I could help them have a career and a future. That career and future can also be short-lived. Hairdressers have to be careful not to let their egos get too overblown. Some hairdressers, when they get busy, become obnoxious and develop this attitude like they're above the law.

Ain't true.

A famous hairdresser named Jean Louie David told me once that when hairdressers start making $1,000 a week because they're so busy, get rid of them. They become a pain in the ass. I don't really believe that. I think that if you understand who they are and what they're becoming, you can deal with it.

Remember: you're only as good as your last haircut.

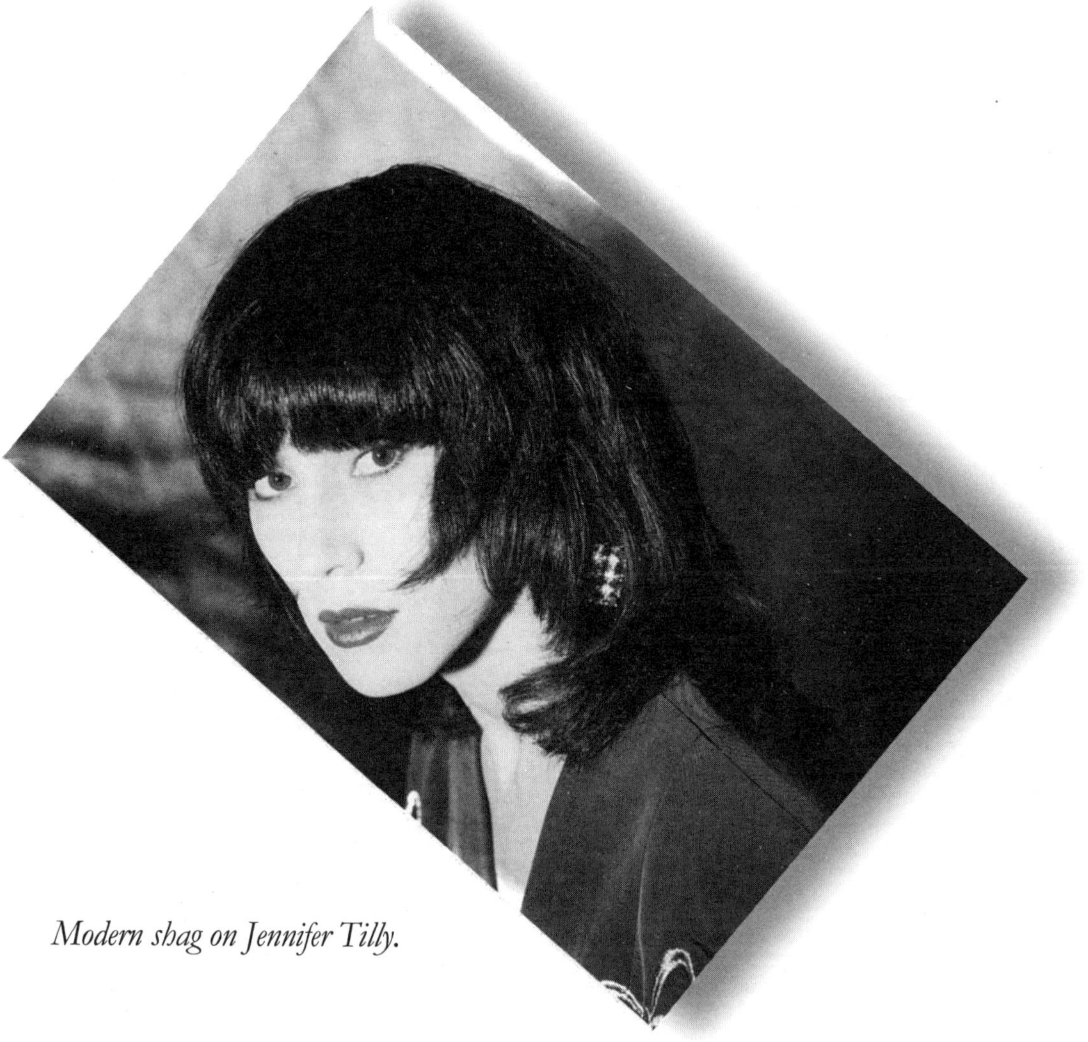

Modern shag on Jennifer Tilly.

It's not just about doing hair. It's about personality and strength. I learned how to be aggressive with a little too much hostility, which worked for a little while—it was sort of the Jon-way of doing things—but it backfired. My hairdressers respected me, but they didn't like me. I actually received hate mail from some of them. That didn't feel good.

I had to learn to trust myself. Just like I had when I was a kid, learning to play the trumpet so that I could rise above my stuttering. When I played the trumpet, I was different. When I took over the salons and they became Allen Edwards Salons, I was different and successful. When I was on stage, I was a god. Things were good. I was learning every day, cutting hair almost every day, fucking my way through life without a care in the world.

It was a crazy way to live. Totally bullshit.

I've always had this dominant personality, and I was learning to control it. I was also smart enough to know whom I could dominate, overpower. I learned how to deal with different personalities. The ones that didn't blend into my life found themselves no longer in my life.

I was the king. Kings get dethroned. But I was going to be king as long as I could.

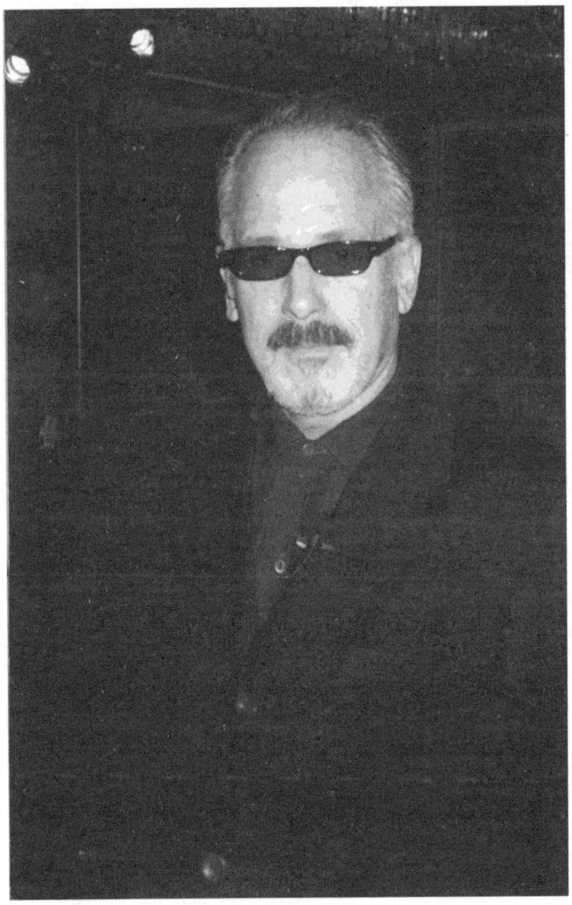

Kings all wear shades at night.

Everything was working. Firing on all cylinders. Since I was so big into cars and motorcycles—the faster, the better—speed ruled my life. I was high on exposure. I never liked drugs. I did try cocaine, and because of my high-energy personality, I could have really gotten into it. I also could have exploded. But I was smart enough not to go that route. Though I did have an addiction to women and sex. What could be more fun?

In those days we called it sport fucking. But I digress.

Everything was working for me because I had great publicity and television exposure. I was on with Regis Philbin all the time. He was my buddy, at least until he went national. People were getting to know me, and that gave me the ability to build people up. It also gave me the ability to tear people down. It gave me power, and power is also a powerful drug.

I lived to be busy. In my salons, I was the hairdresser who did the most people, put through the most volume, made the most money. It also made me feel really good about myself. It gave me confidence. It was my name on the door, after all. It gave me security, both financial and professional. Even if I lost hairdressers, and I did. It's the nature of the business. But I always felt hurt; I took it personally, which made me angry. I still have the reputation that people are afraid to tell me that they're leaving. Instead they just leave. I have the reputation because I have gotten very angry in the past when somebody leaves me. Unfortunately, this has been a difficult thing for me to shake because in my mind, I'm the one who made them. I built them. They're making money and now they don't think they need me anymore. They don't need the education anymore. And I just want to scream, "When you came to me, you were a student looking for a future."

I wonder what I'd be like if I was in the Mafia.

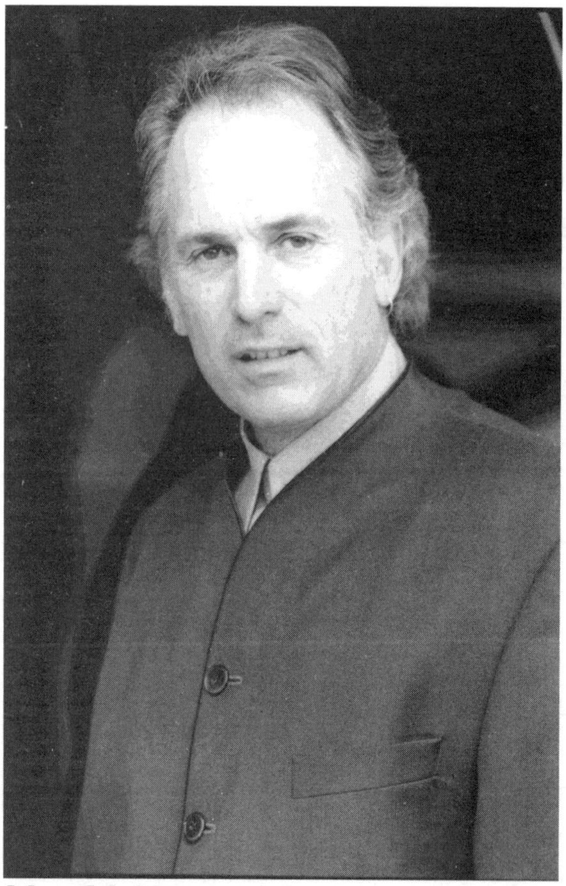

Me as Mafioso.

Most hairdressers are good at leaving but too chicken-shit to sit down and work out a deal. Fuck that.

Hairdressers are all looking for something new and better all the time. They're looking for something different. But when I'd lose hairdressers, I was always able to recover because I was still doing what I do: TV, PR, bringing in clients, recruiting new hairdressers to go on the floor. Hair salons that don't work on their reputation and don't develop a way to bring in new people and new clients end up closing. Not Allen Edwards.

When people do something really well, they can make the mistake of stopping and letting others do it for them. They either expand what they have and are suddenly hailed as this great businessperson, or they stop working and then they go broke.

That's what happened with my partner at the time, Paul Canter. Years after I bought out Jon Peters, the business was thriving, and Paul, who had also been doing hair, decided he didn't want to be a hairdresser anymore. He was going to be a businessman; he became a better golfer. So suddenly the business was supporting him, and I wasn't making any money because it was all going to pay for the business. At the time I was furious. Now I realize that it was my fault for overestimating my partner and my business.

When I first went to beauty school, I loved the constant reinforcement that I got for being good. I think it was about my stuttering. When I was in a situation where I wasn't comfortable, I stuttered worse. But at school, I was good. I didn't stutter. And if I was good inside school, I could be even better outside of school. I was competitive. I was busy. I was a sponge, absorbing everything I could to do more, be better. Rise above.

The Weak Become Strong

Women wanted me. I was a hot commodity. Never mind that I was married. The best thing about being a hairdresser is that everyone loves you and it's a fun, easy way to make money. And I was young and straight. And cute. Even though I've never been tall —5' 6" on a good day—it didn't seem to matter. When you're horizontal, everyone's the same height.

I could be the best hairdresser because there was no such thing as the best hairdresser. Who can say who the best hairdressers are? There are so many talents, so many artistic people. There are lots of bests. Some of the best were Jon Peters, Gene Shacove, Vidal Sassoon, even Geri Cusenza. Many others. They were the best in the 1960s and 1970s and even still today because of their ability to create. I have longevity. This was my education.

But it was draining. The Paul thing was a drain both emotionally and financially. Eventually we parted ways. More on that later.

The biggest drain on me was my father. I was determined that I wasn't going to be like him. He was a great man, but he settled. If he had demons, and I'm sure he did—hell, everyone has demons—he never talked about them. And he never slayed them. Looking at him when I was younger and then as I became successful, I knew that I would never and could never be like him. I couldn't. We shared a gene pool. We wouldn't share the same fate.

When I was a boy, he'd say, "I want to see you drive a Cadillac." So when I first became successful, I bought a Caddy, and then he wanted to know why I spent so much money on a car. He would always find the negative in everything.

That was what drove me forward. It still does. I wasn't going to sit around and wish for more. I wasn't going to live in a house where I was constantly berated. Instead, I would be better, busier, on TV more than ever, do more shows, become more well known. I have an inner drive that's like a high-performance car. All fuel injection and testosterone.

I was good at what I did. I still am. I guess I'm famous (that's what people tell me). I've done a lot of celebrities. Not literally, of course. God knows I tried. But I just did their hair. I used to do Geena Davis' hair. I kind of hinted that I wanted to go out with her. She never came back. I guess I should have stuck to her hair. 5'6" and 6' don't really work.

I know I'm one of the biggest names in the professional beauty industry. Who knows why? It's difficult for me. It's a constant uphill climb, a battle for supremacy at the top for the crown. It's frustrating, but it's what I do. And I love it. I'm always looking for that pot of gold. Waiting for somebody to give me my own TV show. I've always made good money, and everything else is just frosting on the cake. I keep looking for ways to be reborn. I call it the Madonna Syndrome. Keep reinventing yourself and your talent and you keep going forward. (That's why I'm writing this book.)

In the early days there were some celebrity hairdressers who became more famous because of their celebrities. I became famous because of the celebrity hair. It was the work that became famous. The 1970s and '80s were the canvas for my work. It was a canvas that everybody saw because celebrities were on television or on the movie screen; they were on talk shows and in magazines. But to really be a hairdresser, it had to be about the work, the art. The craft.

I love doing hair and dealing with people. I love creating a look and changing a person. I don't care who it is or how old she is. It's about making people feel good because they look so great.

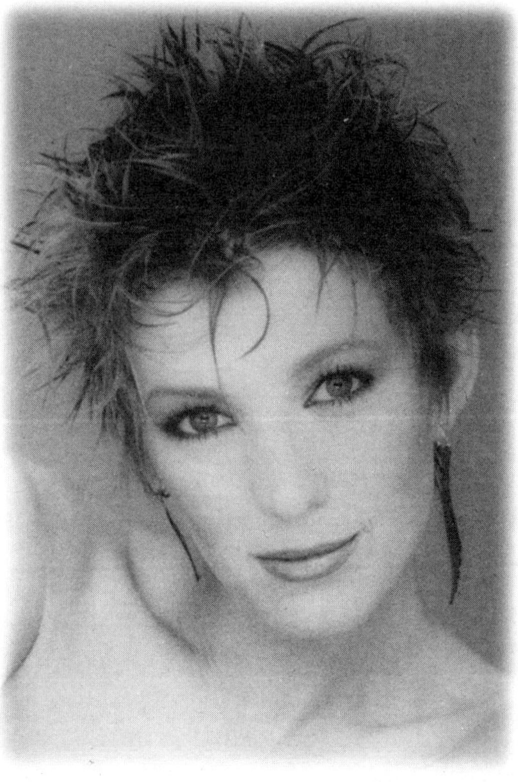

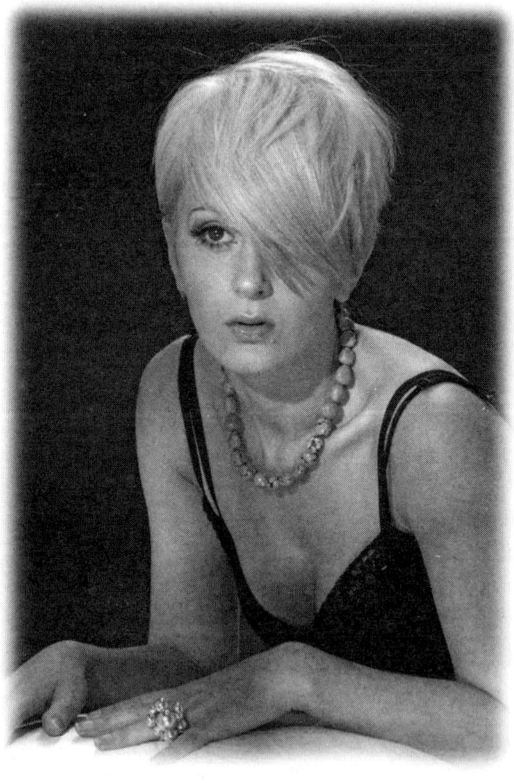

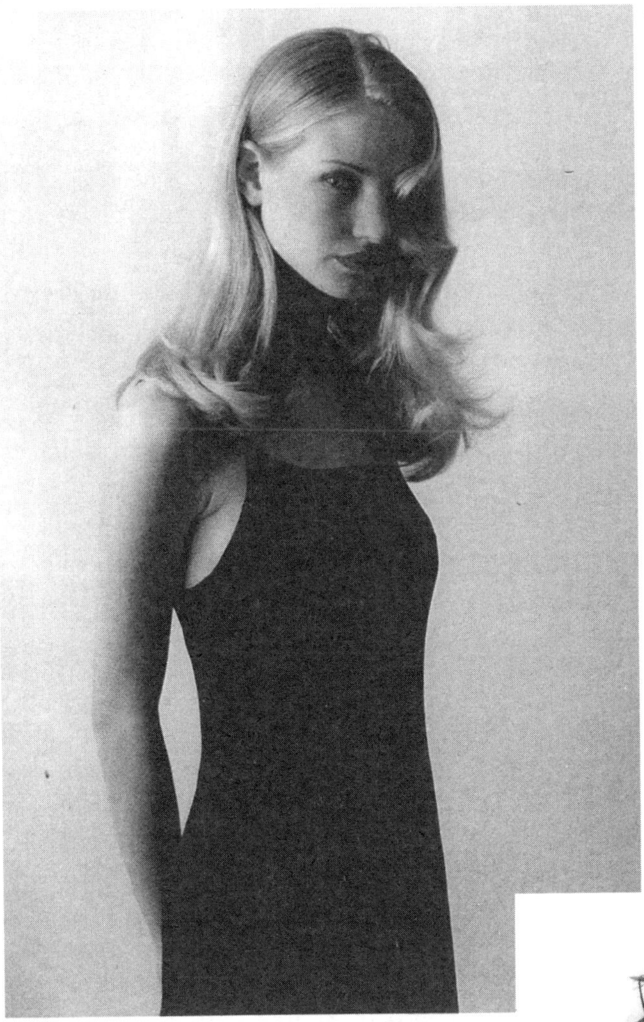

It had to be
about the work,
the art.
The craft.

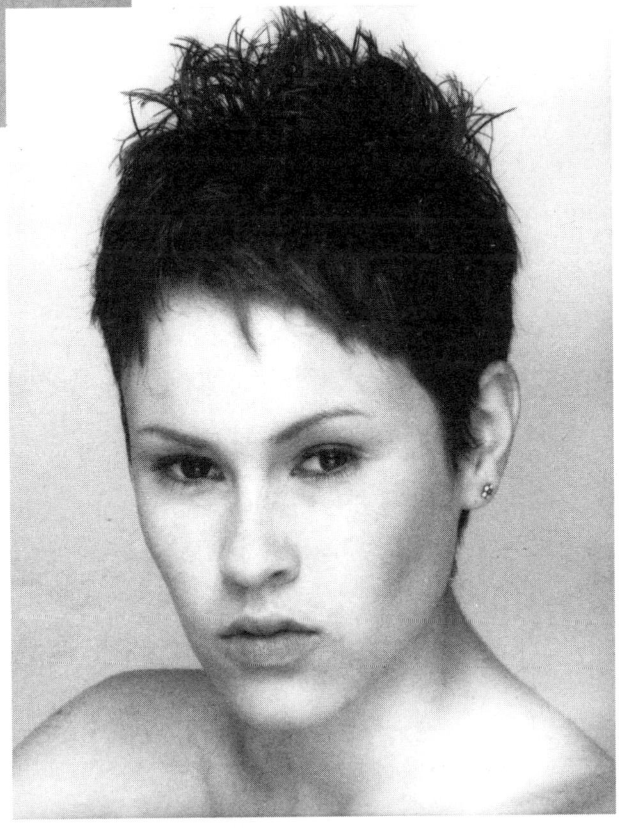

That's the really great thing about being a hairdresser. At the beginning, I had total control over my life and the client's life. I had control over people who were bigger than me, either through their celebrity status or because of their bank account. And I still had control over their lives because I held a pair of shears. It was all about the control. Yeah, and about the work. OK. Fine.

But when I was in control, I didn't stutter.

I could be on stage in front of thousands of people and I didn't hesitate, words didn't catch somewhere between my brain and my mouth. As long as I could control what I talked about—like hair—I was fine.

The roadblocks came when I had to read other people's words. Like reading in class when I was 10 or 11? I didn't have control. It was total panic. Total freeze-up.

That's what happened when a company out of Australia hired me to come over and do a television commercial.

"Allen Edwards? Come on down," said the person on the invisible end of the phone.

"Come on down… where?" I asked, bored.

"Down unda!"

" 'Unda'?"

"Under, under. The land down under, where you tie your wallabies down, sport. We want you to do a telly commercial for SunSilk hair."

Jesus Christ.

Jesus Christ!

A commercial. A telly commercial. A television commercial? Sign me up.

Of course, the whole time flying over there I was terrified. My brain and my mouth were already doing battle. I was looking out the window, seeing nothing but blue sky and blue ocean. Blue on blue, and I was feeling a little blue about what I was about to do.

"You're going to suck," said my brain.

"I can do this," answered my mouth.

"You're going to stutter," said my brain.

"Not if you work with me here," answered my mouth.

"You're going to make a fool of yourself."

"No I won't."

"You'll freeze up. People will point and laugh. You'll never get another job again. You'll become a has-been. A 'hey-isn't-that-that-guy-who-used-to-sort-of-be-famous—' "

My mouth responded: "Hey! I was on Regis. I created the Farrah."

"You didn't do any of those things. I did them."

And my brain was right. It had steered me to near greatness and had helped my mouth to overcome the stuttering. Some people say that stuttering is caused when people think too fast. That might have something to do with it. All I know is that when you start stuttering, the anxiety builds and then you remember you're afraid. And once you're afraid, you're screwed.

I had always been able to overcome my stuttering through sheer force. I knew that if I learned what I was going to say, and it became familiar, I could do it confidently.

You suck—no I don't. As the old Allen was saying, "Holy shit, you're going to have to read," the new, more confident Allen was saying, "I can do this." An epic battle over the Pacific Ocean on a beautiful day in the early 1980s.

I got to the land down unda and was picked up in a limousine fully stocked with more alcohol than I could possibly drink. I opened a Coke and settled into the comfortable seat to observe Sydney from behind blackened glass. It was really a beautiful city. I haven't been back in twenty-plus years, but it had such a young, hip feel to it. It wasn't as set in its ways as some of the older East Coast cities I had played. The people who walked along the sidewalks were very English. Punk was very strong. Hot haircuts, mohawks. It was really happening. They had these huge bags slung low across their chests and onto their hips. They all smoked cigarettes. There was a real sense that great things were going to happen in this city. I actually wanted to stay.

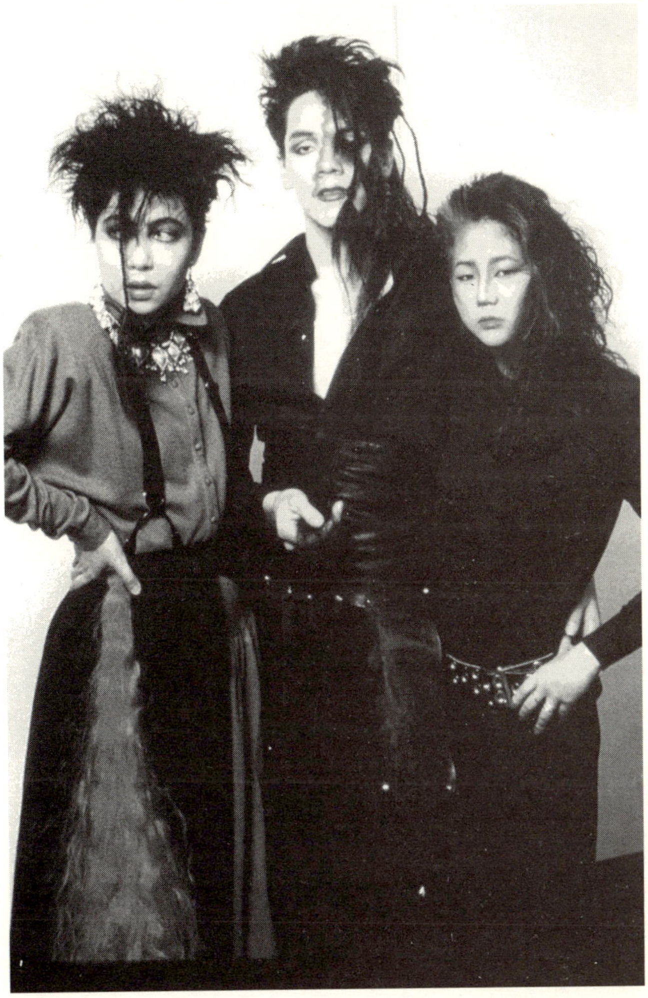

I arrived at my hotel, the Seabell Townhouse. The SunSilk people had booked me into a suite that was again fully stocked with everything my heart could possibly desire. Including the script for the commercial.

Paul was with me. He was like my manager, making sure that everything was the way it should be. He was my rock. He reinforced my greatness, a greatness that was about to come into question.

Television commercials are only 30 seconds long, but this one was all about dialogue and me. I had to learn to memorize. I had to know the material. Hair was my thing, after all. And after reading the script a couple of million times, I knew I was OK. I read it through without a hitch. I even ad-libbed a little. I got hired on the spot to be the spokesperson for four years.

SunSilk was the biggest selling product in all of Australia at the time. They were also very big in Manila. Every four years, they wanted a new celebrity hairdresser to represent the company. Me, being me, wanted to do not only the commercial but also all the hair on the commercial. They let me. I couldn't have asked for anything more stressful.

Back to the commercial. The first one, the first day. I had built up my confidence. I'd be reading great. I'd be flying high. I'd be king of the fucking world and people would want my autograph. Only one problem: I had to say the word "after." But on the first day, I was fabulous.

The second day I was sitting around, waiting for the lighting people. I was seriously considering becoming an actor. Then came the word.

After.

After burn.

Afternoon.

After all.

After. Not a tough word, right? Hell, I said it all the time. But on this particular day, I was in front of the camera and I was talking away and I got to the word.

"aaaafffff."

Silence.

"a-a-a-a-aa-aaa."

CUT.

Complete panic washed over me. I was standing in front of the camera, surrounded by gorgeous models and holding bottles of great goo. I broke out in a sweat. I could feel it running down my back. It was pooling on my upper lip, completely ruining my make-up. It gave me a whole new respect for women.

My confidence was shot. The line was this: "After the rehearsal, the director asked me to get Kate's hair a lot shinier."

"After the rehearsal…"

After my career. Which was ending down unda.

I might as well have been skydiving without a parachute. No one had known I stuttered. It wasn't something I usually advertised, and sometimes I even managed to forget that I did. But I was under the lights, sweating like a pig, the bottles of SunSilk were slipping from my sweaty hands, and I couldn't say the word "after."

"Can I just have a minute?" I said to the director. Notice without stuttering.

Without waiting for approval I went outside. I wanted to throw up.

After. After. After. After. After. After. After. After. After. After. After. After. After.

Then I got an idea. I was going to pretend that the word I couldn't say, the word "after," was the word "dog." And I needed to be moving. So I went back inside, I had a pow-wow with the director. I got my makeup touched up. I got back in front of the camera and my brain was saying "dogdogdogdogdogdogdog-dogdogdogdogdogdogdogdogdogdog-dog-dogdogdog" and my mouth was saying "after" and my confidence level went right back up.

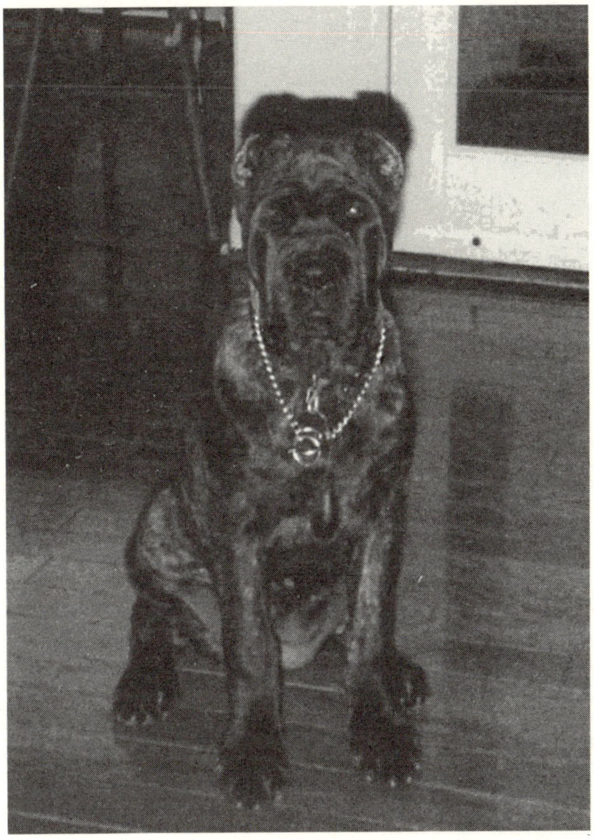

dogdogdogdogdogdog

The commercial was a big success. I'd walk down the street and everyone would recognize me with a nod and a "g'day." I had opened the commercial by saying "Hi, I'm Allen Edwards." The late-night comedians would come out with a bottle of SunSilk just for laughs.

It was great. I felt great. And it gave me some financial freedom. Especially because I had just gotten annihilated in my divorce from Fran.

Yes, Allen. There is a God.

Divorce: Allen style

One of the themes I come across all the time is marriages failing and why it happens. I've had women sitting in my chair for years, women who have gone through many divorces. I'd have one woman sitting in a chair getting a haircut and another sitting in another chair, waiting. The first woman would be talking about her great new boyfriend—who just happens to be the husband of the other woman. Divorce. Isn't it great?

I'd listen to them complain that their husbands didn't understand them, didn't take care of them emotionally or sexually. Their men were never around. I'll always remember this story: one of my clients was talking about having wild sex with her boyfriend. They were in a hotel room somewhere nearby. They rolled over onto her cell phone, which inadvertently dialed the last number she had called, which happened to be her house. The answering machine recorded the whole thing so her husband could hear it when he got home. Can you spell d-i-v-o-r-c-e?

Here's the thing: people get married and then something happens. He gets fat. She stops doing her hair and makeup, stops shaving her legs. They stop being attracted to each other. And then they get divorced. Immediately after that, he drops 20 pounds, she gets waxed from head to toe, and then they're dating other people.

When you're married you have to keep each other turned on visually. It all starts with the visual.

Not everyone looks like Pamela Anderson. Not everyone should look like that. Though *Extreme Makeover* is trying very hard to make it seem like if you go and buy yourself a new head and suck out a new body, then all your problems will be solved. But then you have a whole new problem. What you've become is not really you. It's all artificial. And how do you handle that new person looking back at you in the mirror? How do you respond mentally and physically?

I've had clients who have lost over one hundred pounds but still saw themselves as fat. I hear this is actually quite common.

Anytime you change something on yourself to make you feel better, it's usually a visual change. It can help you grow as a person and give you better self-esteem. If you lose five pounds, you feel better, which motivates you to do something else. Cutting your hair or coloring your hair or trying new makeup is the easiest change you can make. You're trying to look better for you, and maybe for him. Or her.

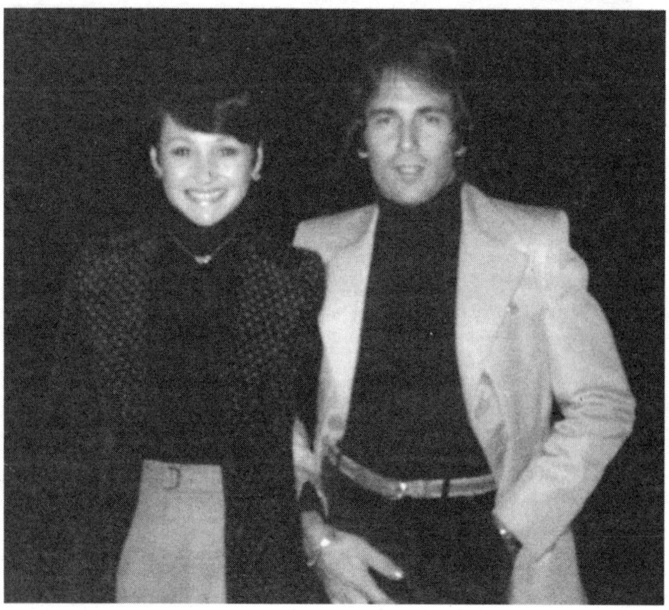

Me and Fran.

But it doesn't always save your marriage. It didn't save mine.

Fran and I probably should never have gotten married. Don't get me wrong. I don't regret doing it. I don't believe in regrets. And if I hadn't married Fran I wouldn't have my kids, Amy and Jason. But we were wrong almost from the start. Hell, we got married primarily so I didn't have to go to Vietnam. That wasn't a great way to start a marriage.

It wasn't just that I was running around, screwing everything. It was that I wasn't any good. I didn't know if our sex was good or bad because I didn't know the difference. We didn't have sex before we got married. But she was a lot of fun even without the sex. She loved motorcycles and fast cars. But after we got married, she changed. Her family didn't approve of me. She was dominated by her sister and her uncle after her mother died, and before dating me she had been in love with a baseball player from high school. She wanted to be married. He moved away, I moved in on her. I was in the wrong place at the right time.

When we first got together, I thought I was supposed to be married. I also rushed into it because of the draft. I did not want to go to Vietnam. We got married, I missed the draft. We had a baby, and I missed the draft again. I thought I loved Fran.

But we didn't work. It was both of our faults.

It might have worked if a number of things had happened. If her mother had lived, if her sister hadn't totally dominated her, if we had moved away. If I hadn't discovered that every other girl I met wanted to go to bed with me. That seemed to have gotten in the way of our relationship. (Can't imagine why.)

A family shouldn't interfere with a marriage. Once a couple is married, that marriage should be off limits to interference. Mom and Dad shouldn't pass judgment. Siblings should stay out of it. Stepchildren shouldn't be the deciding factors.

Fran's family wanted her to marry a professional person, which pushed me to be rebellious. She ended up not liking the business I got myself into, though she loved spending the money.

I was so unhappy. I learned that if you're unhappy in a relationship, you need to get out. You can't subsidize a marriage by cheating, moving or having children. They're never enough to make a marriage work, and in the end, it puts too much pressure on the marriage. More than is already there. It also hurts the children.

It was an interesting phenomenon because I was a boy raised in the '50s. I didn't even realize that you could live with someone and not be married. I was a married man, becoming famous, on TV, cutting celebrities' hair. And believe it or not, I liked being married. I liked that there was someone there even while I was off doing something else, being with someone else.

It's like being a rock musician. I was always looking for the next thing, something better, someone more fun. It's not that surprising, I guess. I was never loyal to a car, to any of my toys. The only thing I was loyal to and truly loved was my profession.

Fran and I went to counseling, which I didn't want to do. I pacified myself by saying that I'd leave later. I'd have lots of girlfriends, sport fuck. Have fun. I look back now and I'm not proud of any of it. I was at the time, but not now. It was an ego trip. Like Bill Clinton getting action under the desk while heads of state waited for him.

My weakness was in not leaving my wife. My biggest fear was living alone. I went from my mother to my wife. In a lot of ways I was no better than Fran. She allowed her family to dominate her, tell her what she should want. I allowed my psyche to dominate me.

So there I was, afraid and insecure. We separated three times, and each time my external life got bigger. I had a bigger home, I had a child and then another. I was having my cake and eating it, too. So clichéd. And so expensive.

Through it all, I never developed any other lasting relationships. I had lots of sex, but nothing that meant anything. All the girls I screwed were married with extremely successful husbands. Stockbrokers, lawyers, doctors. I was out to screw as many women as possible. It was like someone was keeping score, only I'm not sure what the prize was supposed to be.

I never really did drugs. I never courted. I never even went out to dinner. In my mind there was nothing wrong with a haircut and a blowjob. It just happened. Truth: I also never really tried to *not* do it.

There was the Mafia woman. She kept writing me these crazy sex letters while she was under the dryer. She was very sexy. Twenty-seven years old. She wrote about how hot she was, that she was getting wet just watching me work. Her husband was working for John Gotti. One day, this big, black stretch limousine pulled up out in front of the salon and this man who looked too big for even this enormous car got out. He was smoking a cigar and staring at me, like he knew. That time I hadn't even done anything. I was still only, like, 22 years old.

There was the one I called the animal. She was a lawyer's wife. She was 5'8" tall, had a major boob job, exercised her brain away and had a voracious appetite for sex. We met up pretty often.

There was another group of three girls.

I loved sleeping with women who had a lot of money. I think it was my way of getting back at all of the guys in high school who thought they were hot shit and laughed at me because of my stutter. It was the revenge of the nerd.

There was a football player in high school who was always ragging on me. His nickname was Spike. Typical Canoga Park cowboy. 6'1" and 220 pounds. I was doing the hair of this cute little blonde one day and she turned out to be his wife. So immediately, I put on the hustle and ended up sleeping with her. What I didn't realize was that my high school reunion was coming up. I went, in spite of Spike, and he was there. The big fat loser.

Fran and I got divorced.

I fucked around.

I was angry. I was mad at Fran for not wanting to do anything fun—that is, anything I deemed fun. I was angry at myself for getting married. Fran and I had never really gotten along, but my parents didn't get along. I thought that was what marriage was supposed to be. I was angry because we fought all the time. I was angry because I didn't understand the idea of intimacy, even with my wife. I was even angry because of all the sex

I had. I knew I had to clean up my act. There was only so much anger a person could take out on the world by sleeping with anything that moved. Luckily, I met Lisa. We became friends. Eventually we got married. She changed my life.

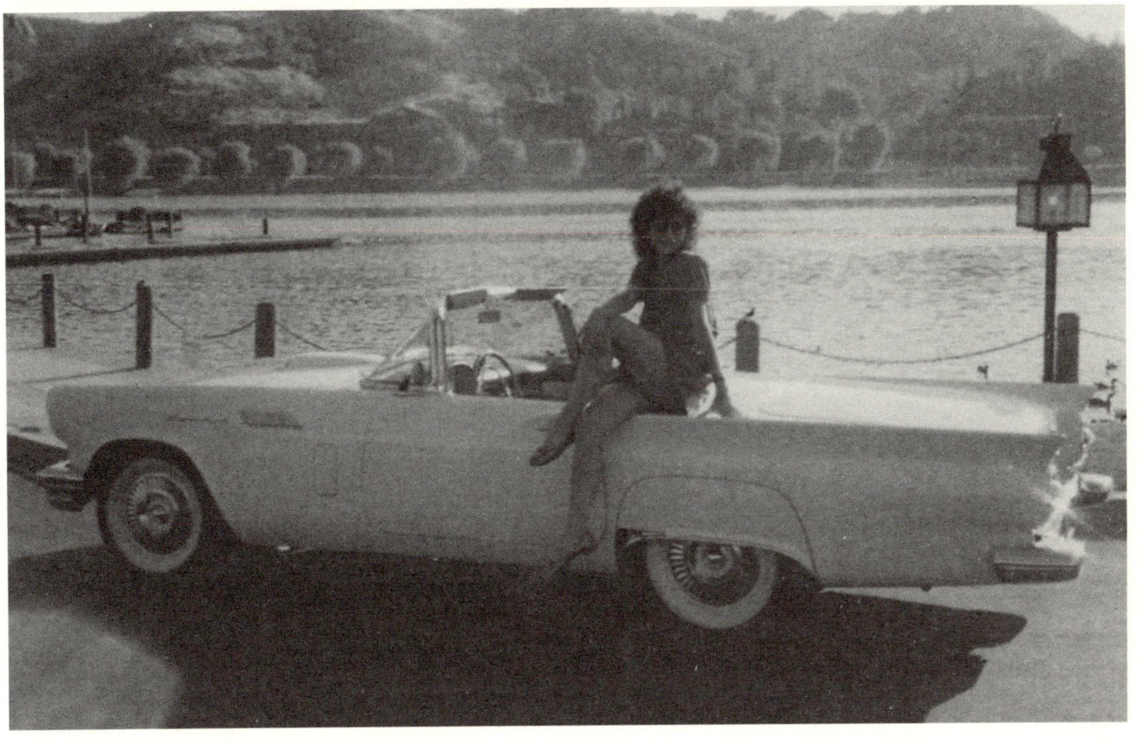

Lisa.

Lisa.

five

Lisa

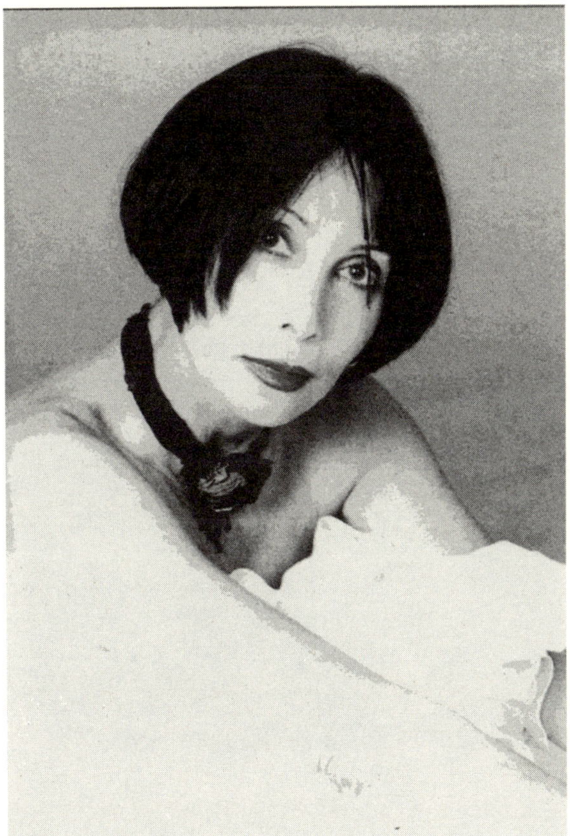

The love of my life: Lisa Edwards.

My first marriage wasn't great, and I was always looking for someone to fulfill what that relationship lacked, namely, total and complete love. One day I was in the salon in Woodland Hills and in walked this Cupie-doll cutie wearing overalls, with a baby on her hip, with long black hair, wanting a new china doll bob haircut. She sat in my chair and all I could think was "what a hot little number." Maybe I could add her to my ever-growing list of conquerees.

But when I looked in her eyes, as she was talking to me about her hair, I got this odd feeling. Usually the feeling I got started just below the belt and stayed there. This feeling started there, and then went directly to my heart. It was a strange and new feeling for me. I didn't quite know what to do with it.

This was my introduction to Lisa. It was the mid-seventies, and both she and I were in our twenties, both in unsatisfying marriages. We didn't act on our desires, even though we both wanted to. Or at least, I wanted to. It was my modus operandi, after all. But instead, we did something different: We became friends instead of lovers. In fact, we all became friends. Fran and Allen and Phil and Lisa. It was the new, more friendly version of Bob and Carol and Ted and Alice, without the swinging. And without Natalie

Wood, even though Lisa bore a strikingly sexy resemblance. [Side bar: I was actually cutting Natalie Wood's hair at the time.]

We'd all hang out together, which was actually pretty easy since we all lived in the same neighborhood in Tarzana. Lisa's husband Phil was very different than me. Very rah-rah college kind of guy. He had a million friends and was very social. He liked to fish and party. He was exactly the kind of guy that I stayed away from in high school and would never, in a million years, have been friends with. But we became friends because of Lisa. Because I got to see Lisa.

So there we all were in our super family suburb where all the up-and-comers lived. We paid $55,000 for a four-bedroom, three-bath house with a yard. Those were the days. Not necessarily the good old ones. In the early days I had tried to buy there, and they wouldn't sell me a house because I was a hairdresser. Hairdresser translated to flakey. The builder was a guy named Norm. I think he was a hunchback.

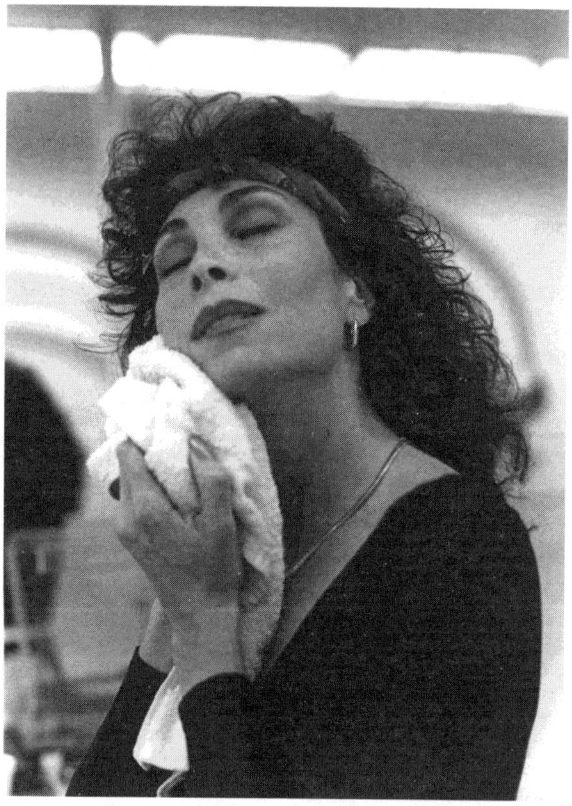

The dancer.

Every time we'd all get together, Lisa and I were glued to each other like Heckle to Jeckle. What bonded us initially was our dancing. She had studied ballet as a kid and still danced. As soon as we'd start to party, Lisa and I would start to dance. We discoed together. I was John Travolta and she was my gorgeous, uptown partner. (It's why I insisted on using her in some of my shows.)

Now granted, I had to play it cool. I couldn't devote all of my time to just Lisa. I did have a wife. I tried to be very cool about my feelings, so I'd hang out with Fran quite a bit of the time when the four of us were together. But I was falling hard. And it wasn't long before I was completely head over heels, nuts in love. I just wasn't in love with Fran.

About once a month we'd all socialize, but Lisa would come to the salon about once a week to "get her bangs trimmed." Honest. We were both totally smitten and absolutely obnoxious flirts, but we had discussed our situation and knew that we couldn't, wouldn't and shouldn't act on our feelings. Damn it.

It would be bad for the kids. I had Amy and Jason and Lisa had Megan.

Hell, it would be bad for our respective marriages. That was new for me, caring about what would happen to my marriage.

This was our life. I'd trim her bangs. We'd all party every fourth Saturday night. And Lisa and I became like two best friends, talking on the phone, laughing together, venting, acting like each other's therapist. Of course, during all of this love and angst, I still kept up with my chosen sport at the time, which was—let's face it—good for my waistline, not to mention my ego.

Speaking of, there was this model I was doing in Beverly Hills, always the last client of the day. Being alone in the salon with her one night, my heart started to pound. She'd sit in my chair and purr softy: "I have no panties on."

"Bul-bul-bullshit."

She proceeded to raise both legs up to the mirror. There it was, the full monkey, staring me in the face. It was the first time in my life I was actually speechless. It took me completely by surprise. She wasn't lying.

Back to real life.

This all went on over the course of several years, during which time my relationship with Fran got worse and worse until I finally decided to leave. Lisa became pregnant at the same time. I moved out, and Lisa and I continued our friendship, but now that I was single, I was wilder than ever, if that was possible. And she was pregnant. With Phil's baby.

I was sowing my wildest oats (not that I hadn't been). I got to experience a three-way, every guy's fantasy. I took two girls and we drove out to Palm Springs for a weekend. Little did I know they were heavily into drugs, one into heroin, the other into high-octane cocaine. I was oblivious. Even if I'd known, I probably wouldn't have cared. All I wanted was both of them. Together. At one time. With me.

We were out at this restaurant one night, and one of them went to the bathroom, leaving me with the other one. I'll call her Jill.

"How's your dinner?" I asked.

"Can't taste it," Jill slurred and I just nodded my head as I spooned pasta into my mouth. I remember '70s pasta was big. Carbs were happening. I needed all the energy I could get. After awhile, the other girl, Jackie, still wasn't back.

"Should we go get her?" I asked. "Should YOU go get her?"

"She'll be back."

And sure enough, as if she had heard Jill's words, which was a physical impossibility, out slid Jackie. She tripped on the flat floor as she came to the table and poured her now coked-out self into the chair. I continued to eat my pasta and Jill started to laugh. Loudly. That made me laugh, too. And then Jackie was laughing as well, flat-out hysterical. The whole restaurant crowd was watching us. All the blue-bloods out in Palm Springs for a weekend of golf and relaxation, all looking at the freaky hairdresser with his long hair and his two women.

Two women. It still makes me smile.

Next thing I knew, Jackie did a face-plant into her plate of pasta. It was spaghetti and meatballs, if memory serves. The meatballs rolled off the plate and onto the floor. It was like a scene out of a movie. Everyone was looking at us. The restaurant was totally silent. You could hear ice melting in the glasses. And neither Jill nor I knew what the hell to do.

"We can't leave her like that," Jill whispered as she leaned over to me, exposing her ample cleavage and giving me a hard on.

"Well. Maybe she's just really hungry," I offered. "Maybe after she's done doing whatever she's doing, she'll be ready to go."

"She won't be able to walk," Jill whispered. I could feel her breath on my face and on my arms. The hair on the back of my neck was standing at attention. So was something else.

I did the only thing I could think of. I stood up, I pulled Jackie's face out of her food, picked her up and carried her out of the restaurant. Jill took my cue and ran ahead of me, opening the doors to the restaurant and to the car so that I could dump Jackie in the back, which I did. Then off we went to the hotel.

Like I said: Wild.

This kind of sporting went on for about eight months, but during the whole time I was still thinking about Lisa. So what did I do? The only thing a red-blooded, American hairdresser could do. I went back to Fran. Surprisingly, she actually took me back.

I stayed with her and my kids for two more long, grueling years. My friendship with Lisa grew even stronger. She was special. Not that the girls in Palm Springs weren't special. They were just a different kind of special. They were weekend special.

Lisa was lifetime special. Even when she got sick years later, she was special. I had never believed in soulmates, but with Lisa, I knew that she was the last woman I would ever be with. Would ever want to be with. She completes me. Even in the 1970s I was smart enough to know that.

Lisa had another baby girl. I started having fantasies about taking her out on a real date. But she was still married and I had moved back in with my wife. We were both unhappy, me especially.

So what do you do when you're miserably frustrated with your relationship? Buy another house. Of course.

Fran and I packed up the kids and moved to another neighborhood in Tarzana, across the street from Sally Field. It was a Cape Cod that had been redone, and it sat on a half acre of land. Huge in Los Angeles. Jason, my son, was five. My daughter Amy was ten. I was miserable and building a master bedroom that I didn't really want.

After months of dealing with contractors and designers and making trips to the hardware store, we were finally ready to finish the bedroom. It had six French doors and hardwood floors. The ceiling was vaulted. It was absolutely spectacular. Gorgeous. A room anyone would want to live in.

I stood in the doorway and looked at what I had created, and I realized that I was done. Done with the room, done with the marriage. I had spent all my time trying to refurbish my bedroom, and what I was really trying to do was rebuild my marriage. It didn't work. It was time to move on.

Even though I wanted to stay for my kids, I knew that was a mistake. People stay together so often for the wrong reasons. This was one of those really wrong reasons. I truly should have left long before this, even before Lisa. I was staying in a marriage I didn't want to be in, screwing around, and being unhappy. Coming up with all kinds of reasons not to leave. As a hairdresser I always heard about people being afraid. Women were afraid to leave because they didn't know what their rights were; men didn't want to give up half of everything. If you can get past the fear, life flourishes. You wouldn't keep a dog that kept biting you. Why keep a husband or wife you don't like? I also knew that both Amy and Jason would ultimately be better because they would be in a better environment, a happier environment.

I walked out that day for the last time.

I immediately got myself a condominium and started redoing that. That's the flamboyant side of me. Decorating.

A month later, Lisa left Phil.

My life was about to take a new and interesting turn, and I couldn't wait.

Now, imagine the timing of all of this. Both of us leaving our spouses at roughly the same time. For a long time we had kept our feelings quiet, and now we had both left our respective spouses within a period of two months. We had a very long, very serious discussion and knew that we needed to be together. I had already spent years fantasizing about Lisa being by my side. I used to fantasize even when I was with Fran. Once I even said Lisa's name. Fran turned to me and asked, "What did you say?"

I came up with some flimsy excuse.

We went to a dance recital once where Lisa was performing, and I was way too excited for what it actually was. I even brought flowers.

"Are you fucking her?" Fran asked me on the way home.

"Are you kidding?" I said. "She's too skinny for my taste." (Not really.)

Truth be told, Lisa and I couldn't imagine our lives without each other. It was a primal need.

We both filed for divorce, no separations necessary. Certainly not on my part. I'd already been down the separated road, and I knew what path to choose. And we started dating. *Finally.* Can you hear the sigh of relief in that word?

It wasn't too long before Fran found out, and she went absolutely ballistic. The saying "hell hath no fury like a woman scorned" was invented for my soon-to-be ex-wife. But the scorn was largely perceptual. I hadn't left her for Lisa. I had left because of me, and because Fran and I just didn't work. Still, the other saying that exists for a reason is "perception is reality." I wasn't stupid enough to fight her when she went after everything. Luckily my lawyer was smarter, and we came to what I thought was a fair agreement. She got the house, and alimony for nine years (this on top of the two years I'd been paying her since we filed for divorce). We both got the kids, joint custody. I got my freedom. After 10 years of marriage.

A year after leaving Fran for the third and final time, Lisa and I moved in together. We bought a house in Encino, down the street from Phil Hartman, the late comedian whose wife eventually shot and killed him. In retrospect, I got the better deal.

My kids were not happy at all. I was living with someone who wasn't their mother, living with someone else's kids. I think they felt that I had chosen Lisa's kids over them. That couldn't have been further from the truth. It was something both Amy and Jason eventually realized, but it took us a long time to get there. At the time they felt their father had abandoned them. I hadn't. But that was their perception and their reality.

I tried to include them in my new life. I would see them for an extended weekend every week. Sick or not. We all played big, happy, dysfunctional family. We had fun Fridays where we'd go to the movies, all of us. But my kids wouldn't sit behind Lisa in the car. So it went.

There was a lot of door slamming by Amy and sulking by Jason, mainly because of the door slamming by Amy. Jason thought he was supposed to hate me and my new life. He

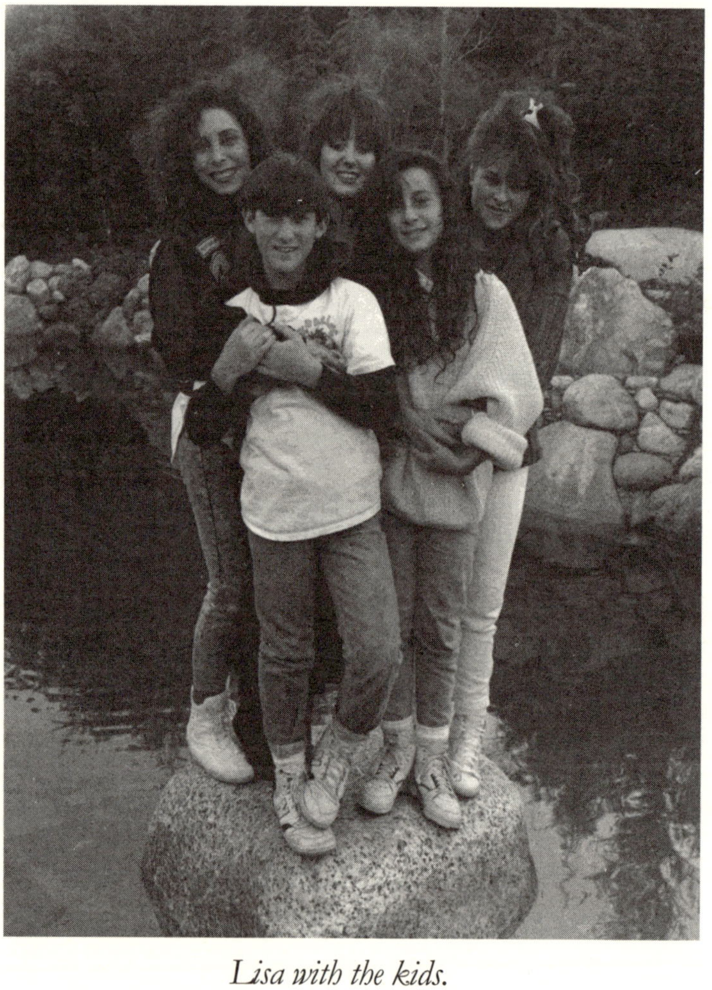

Lisa with the kids.

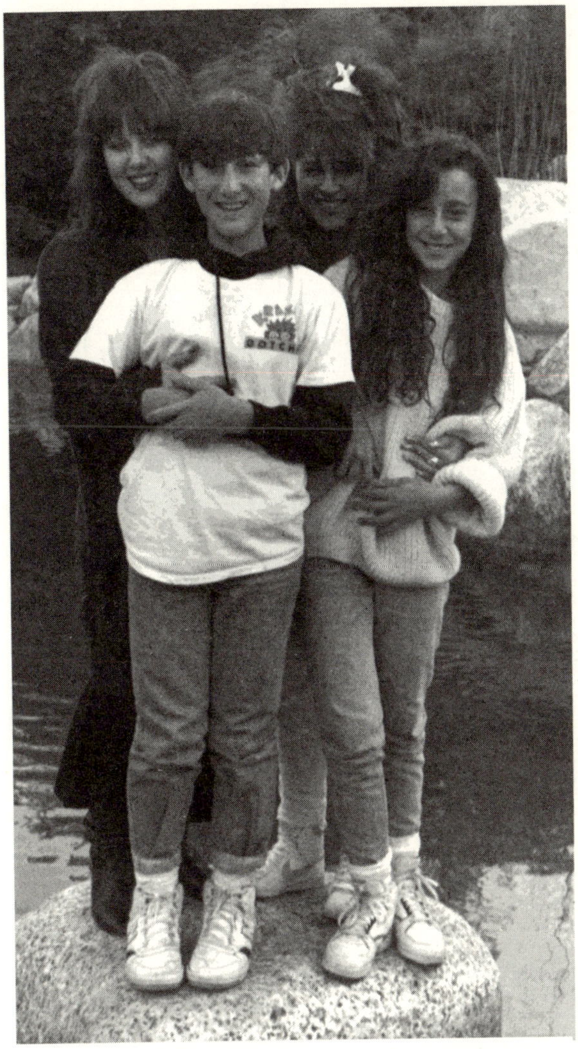

The kids: Hers and mine.

took his cues from Amy. I understood. It was hard. It was asking them to do a lot. To basically accept that their father, who had almost always been in their house with their mother, was now living in another house with two other kids' mother.

It was stressful on us all, but if anything good had come from my marriage to Fran, it was my two kids. I would do anything to help this situation. I would give my life, my career, my everything for my kids. It's a cliché, I know. If you have kids, you understand. They are part of me. They are half of me. I love them more than my own being.

I had two friends, both divorce lawyers. They both left their wives and in essence divorced their kids, too. I thought that was disgusting and weak.

It took seven years before we were finally a family. It was a long seven years.

A year after Lisa and I moved in together, we got married, on September 28, 1980. We had a country-western wedding at our new house. A big hoedown on the front lawn. We even made the rabbi wear a cowboy hat. We had pie instead of cake. Everybody had to come in western wear. My ex-partner Frank showed up in a limo wearing a full Indian headdress down to the floor.

Sixty people got drunk to country-western music, me included.

I kept being John Travolta. First I was *Grease* when I was a kid. Then I was Tony Manero in *Saturday Night Fever*. Now, at my wedding, I was wearing a cowboy hat like in *Urban Cowboy*. All these years I thought I was Steve McQueen. How the hell did I become John Travolta? And who am I really?

On our wedding night, we went to a hotel downtown. I was pretty intoxicated. I decided to wake myself up with a line of cocaine. Me, the non-drug guy. I threw up even though I was wired like an electrical unit. Needless to say, our wedding night was NOT one of our best nights.

Our wedding day was one of the happiest of my life, and one of the most fun. Yee-haw!

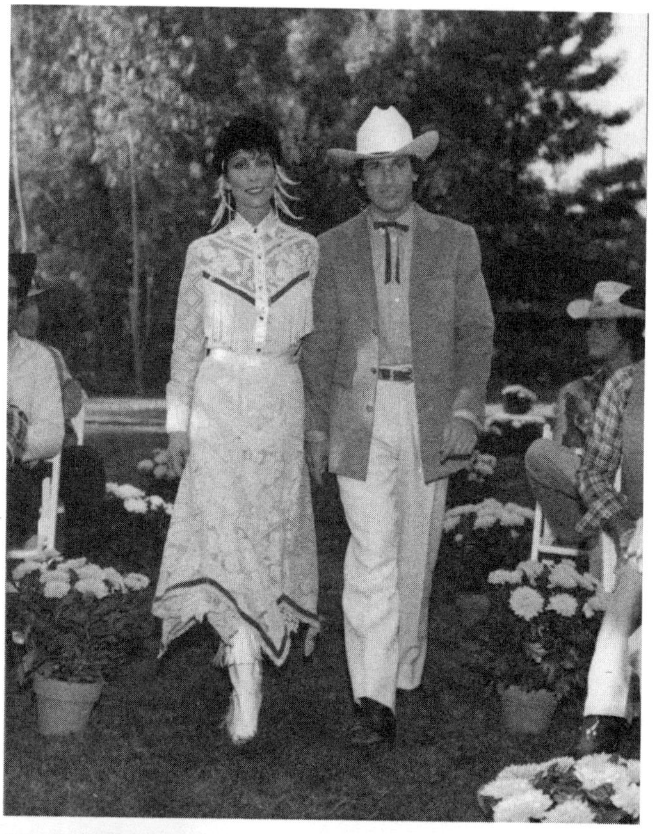

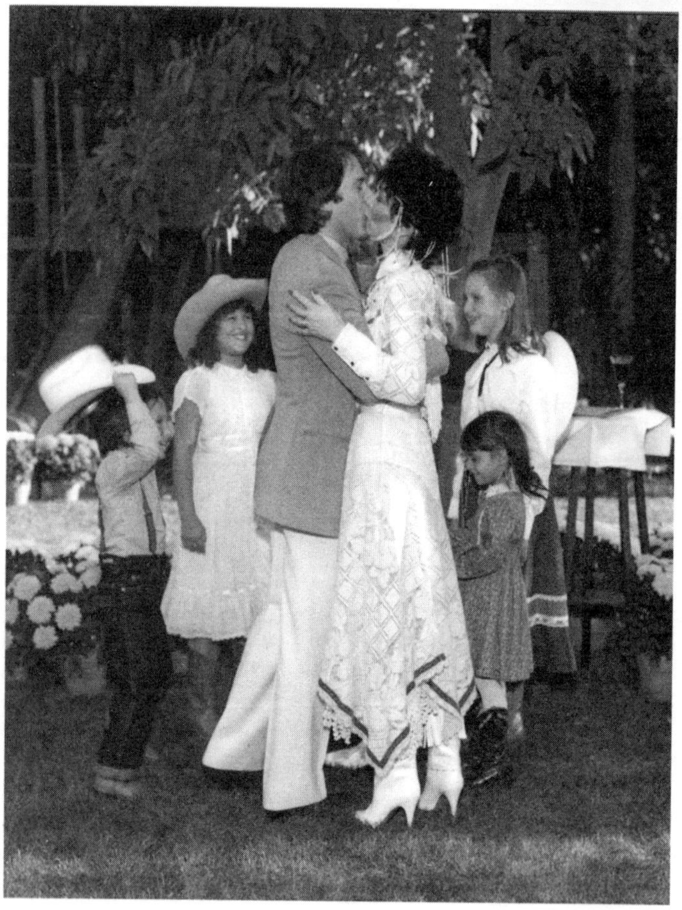

I now pronounce you husband and wife and kids.

It was right around this time when I first hit on an analogy for my life. I'm sure I wasn't the first one to think this, but it was new to me nevertheless. My life was like a game of Monopoly. I had game pieces that I moved around the board after I rolled the dice. I'd roll a two and my kids would come for the weekend; a six and they'd stay for a week. Sevens meant that Lisa and I would do just fine. When I rolled and the dice flew off the board, signifying a re-roll, I knew that I was in trouble. That happened a lot.

When my obligation to pay alimony was finished, all eleven years of it, the attorneys had left a window open that allowed Fran to take me back to court. She did. She wanted alimony for life. I had remarried, and she was pissed off.

Fran hired Arlene Coleman Schwimmer, a shark of an attorney. I swear I saw her black eyes roll back into her head every time we were in court. She was a ball-buster. She was also David Schwimmer's mother. David Schwimmer would eventually go on to pop culture fame as Ross Geller on NBC's breakthrough angst comedy *Friends.*

Going back to court to rehash my marriage and the alimony was like being in jail for nine years and finally getting out, only to be told that the law had changed and now I had to go back to do a life's term.

Crap.

I remember going to the courthouse one day, knowing that my financial fate was about to be decided once again. There was a homeless guy who hung out near one of the trees, under the shade.

"Man, can you give a brother some money?" he asked.

"Buddy," I said as I stopped to talk to him, "I have a feeling I might be sitting next to you soon."

I walked into the courthouse.

I walked out having agreed to pay my ex-wife even more money. In the courthouse, when it was my lawyer's turn to speak, I looked up and the judge was falling asleep. I knew my life was over. Fran had tried for lifetime alimony. She didn't get it. But she did get another lump sum of $50,000.

Men, listen up: when you're getting divorced, try to settle as fast as possible. The longer it goes, the longer you pay the lawyers, and the crazier it gets. In the beginning of a divorce there are still some feelings there. She might still care a little. Damned little. But the longer it goes, she could end up turning into an ax-murderer. Get out quick.

That was the last time I had to pay Fran. It was the true beginning of my freedom from my old life. I lost a lot of money on that marriage. But I left with my name. My name was my calling card.

Now all I had to deal with was the coming apocalypse of AIDS, and the implosion of my business. Good times for sure.

Good times for sure.

six

Allen as metaphor

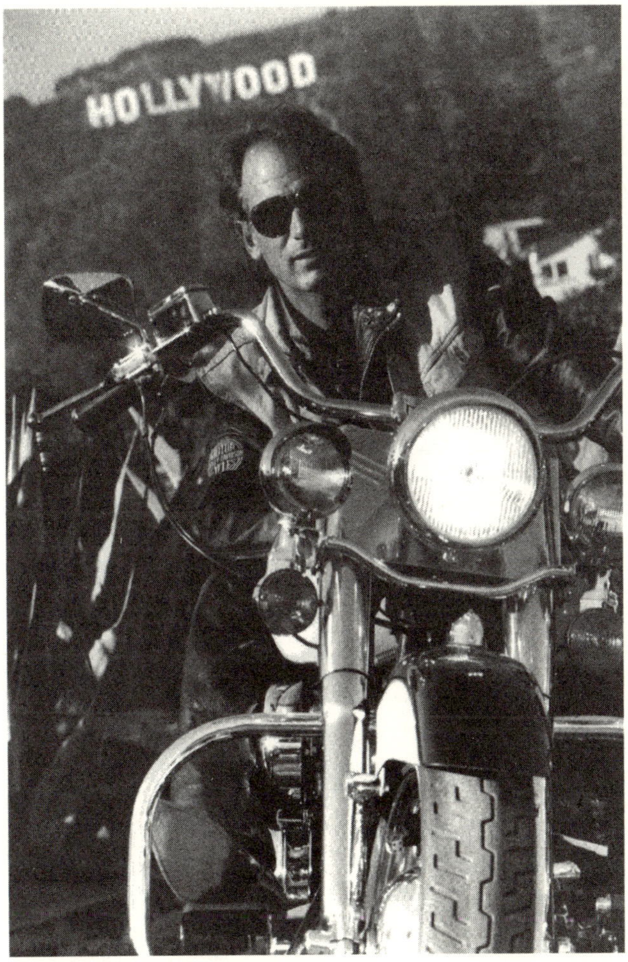

I got arrested on my motorcycle once. Every young Jewish man should always get arrested on his motorcycle at least once. It's good for the soul.

I was having a particularly bad day at the salon. I had lost some hairdressers and was stressing out. I did what any red-blooded American, heterosexual hairdresser with an attitude would do. I got on my Harley and drove to Malibu. Through the winding, twisting Topanga Canyon I cruised, just so I could get a cup of coffee at this great diner. The ocean was glistening. It calmed me down immediately. I felt better just feeling the sea air on my face and the wind in my hair. I had hair then.

On my way back into the Valley, on Las Virgenes Road/Malibu Canyon, one of the coolest roads to ride on a bike, there was very little traffic, lots of open road. I don't even think I was speeding. All of a sudden there was this siren, and in my mirrors, a cop. (Shit!) I pulled over and he decided to harass me.

I'm sure I had a slight attitude problem. Slight. Like my stutter, which was strangely non-existent that day, at least at first.

"What'd I do?" I asked as he put me up against the car, hands splayed on the hood (which was hot, can I just say) and started patting me down like I was some kind of criminal.

"Your pipes are too loud," he growled.

"My pipes. Are too loud?" Now I knew he was full of shit. My bike was kind of radical, especially for the time: raked out, blacked-out chrome. It was way ahead of its time. But I also knew he couldn't even see my pipes from the angle we were at, let alone hear them. "Then you must stop just about every biker you see, 'cause nobody, and I mean nobody, has stock pipes."

He asked to see my license and registration. I pulled out my wallet.

"Your license is expired," he said. Things were going from bad to worse.

"Yeah, well, about that," I started.

"So's your registration." This was almost too embarrassing to tell.

"Yeah, well, I-I-I—"(breathe). "I ha-ha-have an appointment. At the DMV. To-to-tomorrow." My dog ate it.

"Tomorrow," he said rather than asked. He didn't believe me.

"Too much?" I said as he spun me around.

"Too much," he said. He confiscated the bike and put me in the back of the squad car. This is the best part. He actually asked me if I had stolen the bike.

"What?" I asked. I'm Allen Goldstein, nice Jewish hairdresser from the Valley. How could I steal a bike? "No."

He got in and peered at me from the rearview mirror.

"I probably should have said I have an appointment, like, next week, huh?" I said from the back seat.

"Might've been a little less obvious," he grumbled from the front seat as he drove me back into the Valley.

I was quiet for a while, watching the scenery go by, scenery I should have been enjoying ON MY BIKE.

I decided to invoke the charm offensive.

"So. You married?" I asked innocently from the back seat.

"What the fuck are you asking me that for?" he said. He was mad, like, how dare I even ask such a question (buddy, I know more about wives than you could ever know).

"It's just that I have hair salons," I said.

"Hair salons."

"Yeah. In Woodland Hills, Encino and Beverly Hills. You should have your wife come see me sometime." Always looking for more business. Maybe she could get a makeover. I could put her on Regis. I could just see it: The cop's wives makeover show. And then I could get him back by sleeping with her.

"Why would I do that?" he asked.

"Because I'm offering," I said with a shrug.

He nodded and kept on nodding as we twisted our way back to the Valley. At the corner of Ventura and Topanga Canyon, right before one of the busiest intersections in the West Valley, he pulled over. And he sat there, staring straight ahead. I was thinking, he's going to shoot me.

Finally, he got out of the car and opened the back door. I peered out at him.

"OK, Edwards. Get out," he said.

Now I started thinking that he wasn't going to shoot me; he was just going to beat the crap out of me. Right there. In the West Valley. In front of a telescope shop. I was just hoping that someone inside had his or her lens trained on us. I needed a witness.

"Get out of here," he said.

"Wh-what?"

"Go on. You can pick up your bike tomorrow." I got out, he got back in and drove away. I stood there, rubbing my wrists, trying to figure out just how the hell I was going to get home. Maybe I should call my mommy.

Hard core biker guy. That was me. Right.

Years later, I got to experience what it was like to be a real biker type. My bike mechanic and I had become good friends. He invited me to go up into the local mountains around Los Angeles with him and two of his buddies. There were no helmet laws at the time. I suited up in my ripped Levi's, my biker boots, a leather vest and a bandana. Off we went.

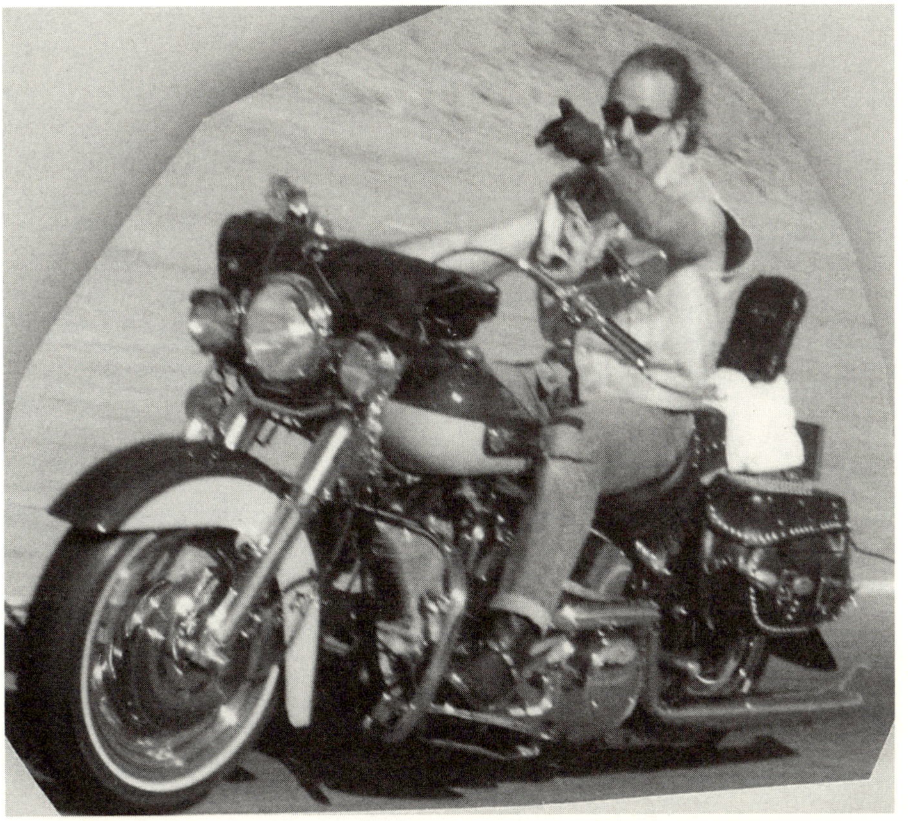

It was summer. Going through the desert on the 10 freeway, through what's known as the Inland Empire, it was about 100 degrees. As we climbed up into the mountains, it dropped into the low 40s. We stopped along the road to put on our leathers and continued. The sun became the moon and nighttime brought out the biggest bugs I'd ever seen. We're talking horror movie size. Like *Them.* And I had to scrape them off the front of my bike. It's part of the biker experience. I looked like John Travolta (again) in *Road Hogs*, picking these animals out of my teeth. Sexy.

We went to Chad's bar, up in Big Bear. It was the next day, the day after the bug fest. The three guys were drinking. I wasn't much of a drinker. But if you're gonna ride with the big dogs you gotta pee on the big trees, whatever the hell that means. They were downing beer and shots, boilermakers, like water. I had one. I was a pussy. They didn't seem to notice.

Then we went to this biker bar called Hog Heaven. It was the epitome of a biker bar. Kind of redneck. Wooden planks, neon signs screaming beer, a split rail fence where cowboys used to tie their horses and dudes now parked their hogs. We walked in and immediately I saw these two 8-foot-tall bikers standing in front of me with their arms crossed over their barrel chests. I felt like I was in a biker movie. I was cool. I did the biker nod. You know, the barely imperceptible chin drop and rise. Eye contact. (Don't beat me up.) No smile.

The place was full of bikers and girls. They were playing "Wild Thing" on the jukebox. Then "Born to be Wild." The bartender was a girl. She was missing three teeth. (This was one I didn't want.) I leaned over the bar and she leaned toward me. Our faces were about an inch apart. She smelled like tequila.

"Whadaya have?"

"A diet Coke," I whispered. "It's a little late for me." She snorted but shoved a glass across the bar at me.

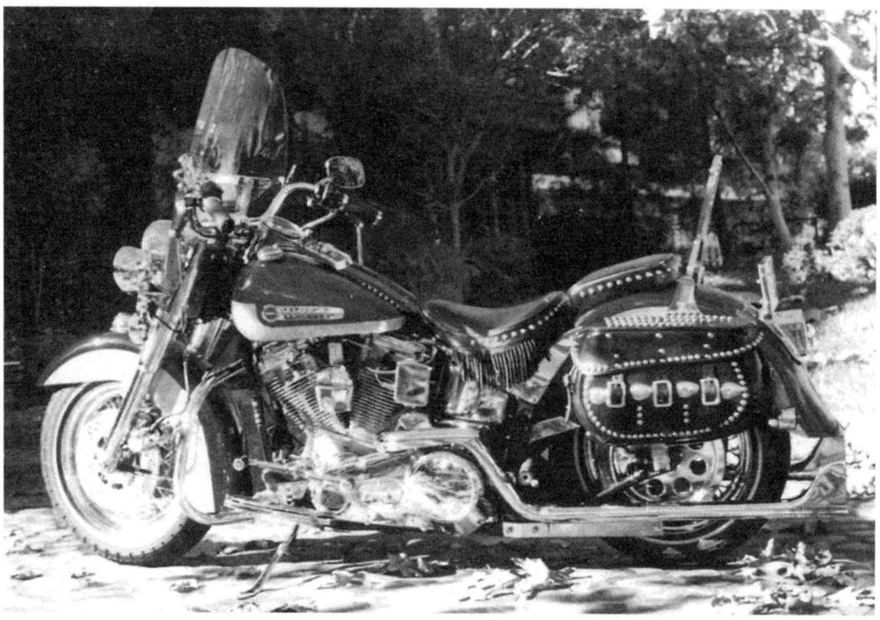

I was panicking a little, thinking that one of the other guys was going to ask me what I did for a living. I leaned against the bar, sipping on my Coke. I decided I was a bounty hunter. Maybe I owned a garage. Anything other than being a hairdresser. It wasn't very macho. Not in a biker bar called Hog Heaven.

I walked outside. This 300-pound biker, a big dude, was walking toward me. I was standing near my bike, thinking, "How fast can I fire this thing up and get out of here?" Not very. The bike was parked nose in, which meant I would have to get on, start it up, back up, kick it into gear. Too long. I was going to die.

"Nice ride," the guy says.

We bonded right there in the parking lot. The skinny Jewish hairdresser from the Valley and a guy who was about the size of a Chevy. His name was Tiny. No kidding.

All I could think was back when I was a kid, seeing that guy on the bike who was so cool. Now I had the best of all worlds. I was the cool biker (drinking diet Coke) on the weekends and a mild-mannered (yeah) hairdresser surrounded by hot women all day.

Hey. Somebody had to do it.

So this was my life. I was a hairdresser, I had successful salons. I was a rock star on stage. I wrestled with my stuttering. I was a husband, a father, a business owner. Life was good.

It was the 1980s. Things were starting to change. My wife was starting to get ill, and we didn't know what was wrong. I was losing some of my closest friends and colleagues to the "gay plague," AIDS. And I was worried about looking butch in a biker bar.

Allen. Meet metaphor. Let's get our priorities straight here.

Life Was Good

My life was fun. I admit it. I liked my life. I had great kids. I was finally married to the woman I loved. The woman who completed me. I loved my job. I had cars, boats and motorcycles. We had a great house. Life was good.

We even had dogs. I'm going to digress for just a minute because dogs have always been important to me. They have this ability to take me away from women, from colleagues. From stress. They're just who they are. They don't care what I do for a living, if I have a big house or an expensive car. They ground me. They keep me in touch with who I am.

The more different they are the better. I think it has something to do with my distorted ego. I love the attention I get when everyone stops me to ask what kind of dog that is. They never wonder who I am. Somehow that's OK.

Too many people get dogs for the wrong reasons. Like they're a fashion accessory. That's why there's the joke about people looking like their dogs. I've had Great Danes, miniature Dachshunds, Akitas, chows, every kind of dog you could imagine. People look at little puppies and coo—"Isn't it sweet?"—and then it grows up to be this humongous Rottweiler. They wanted a cuddler and they ended up with a hunter, a guard.

Allen Edwards

Dogs are my alter ego. I suspect I like rare, big dogs because they're more of a challenge to deal with. I've had a Neapolitan Mastiff. I've had a Cane-Corso, an 85-pound chow, a 110-pound pit bull. I love when I get asked, "Why do you have that dog?" And I always answer, "Because I can." I even got involved with protection training at one point.

My dog, Blade, is a pit bull. He has a head the size of a small boulder. He is the most affectionate and needy of any dog I've ever owned. I lose sleep over him sometimes, he's so good. So real. But even I know you don't want to mess with a pit bull. He's still what he is.

Dogs are real.

My new Cane-Corso pup, Kiante.

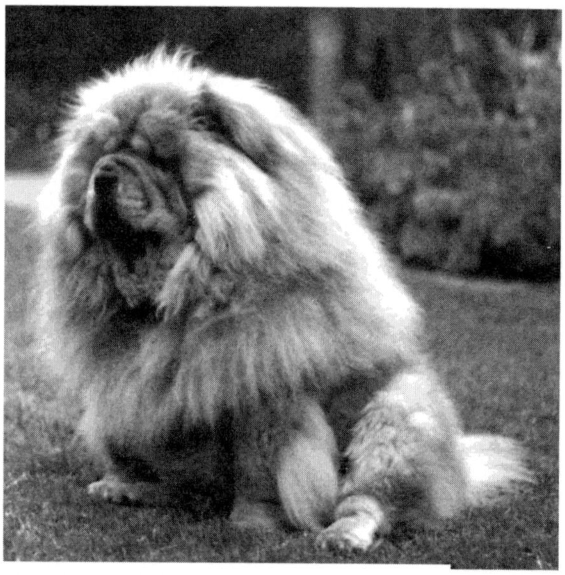

My beloved chow, Kanzi.

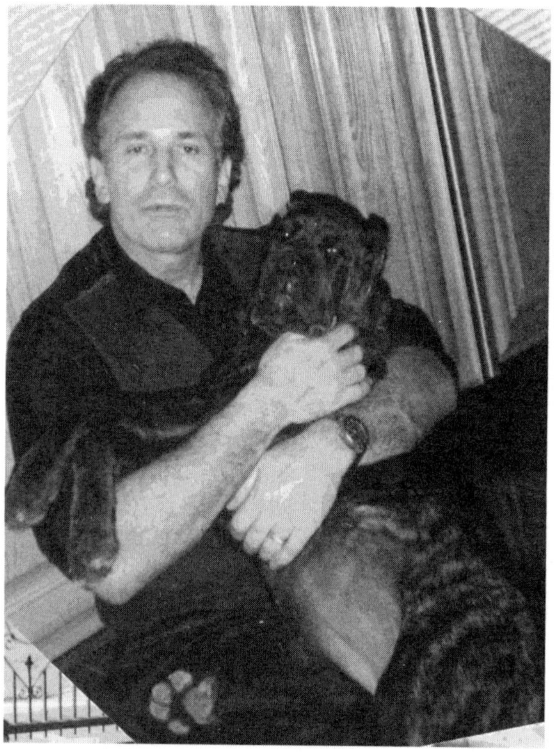

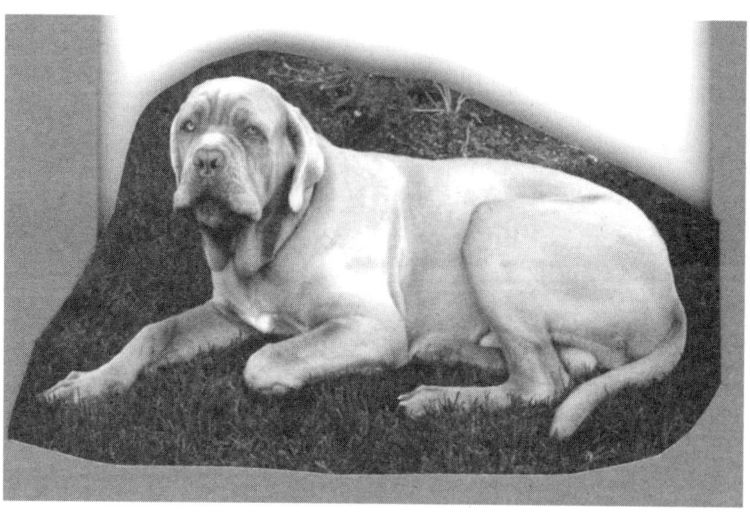

Enzo.

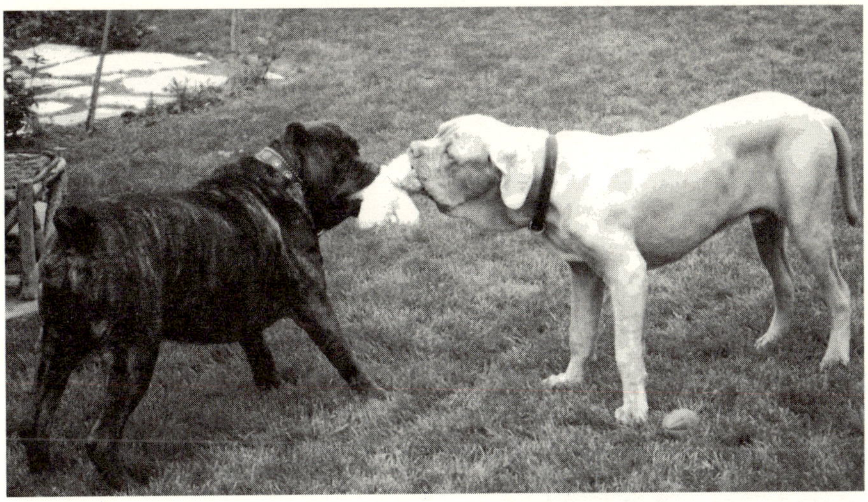

Enzo and Kiante.

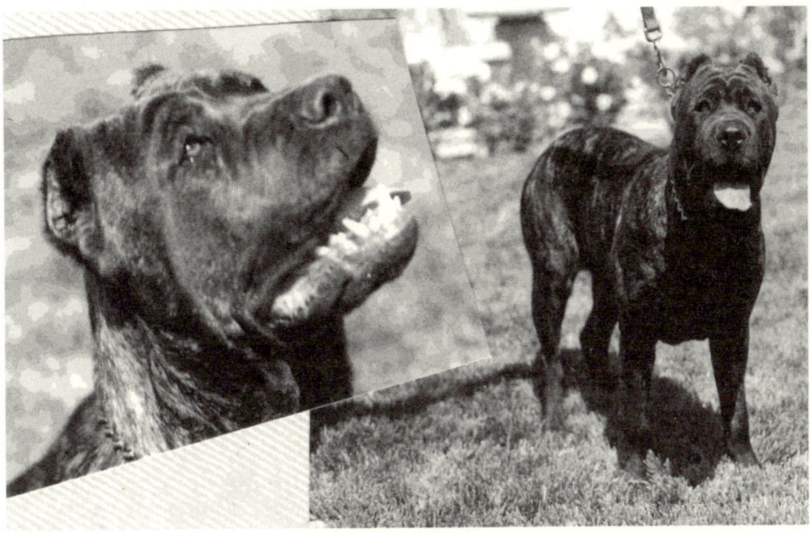

Dogs are real.

Kiante.

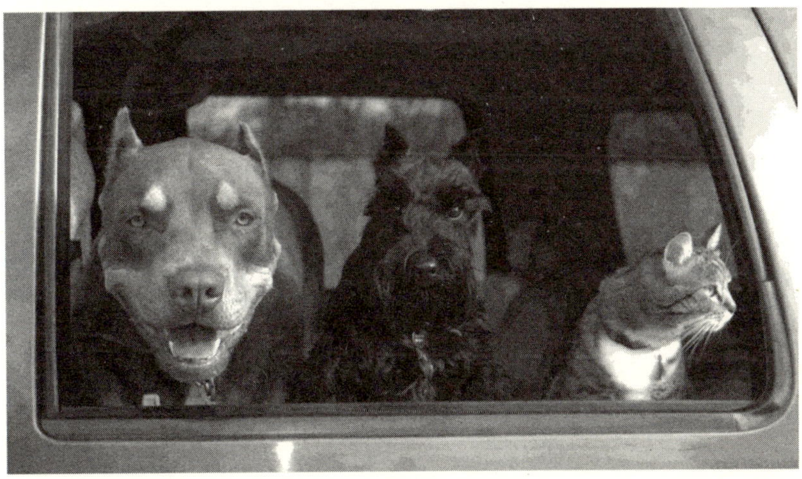

Blade, Parker and Montana.

Dogs are life. I think that's why they have always been so important to me, and why I need them in my life. They ground me, especially when things start going bad. And in the 1980s, they started going bad.

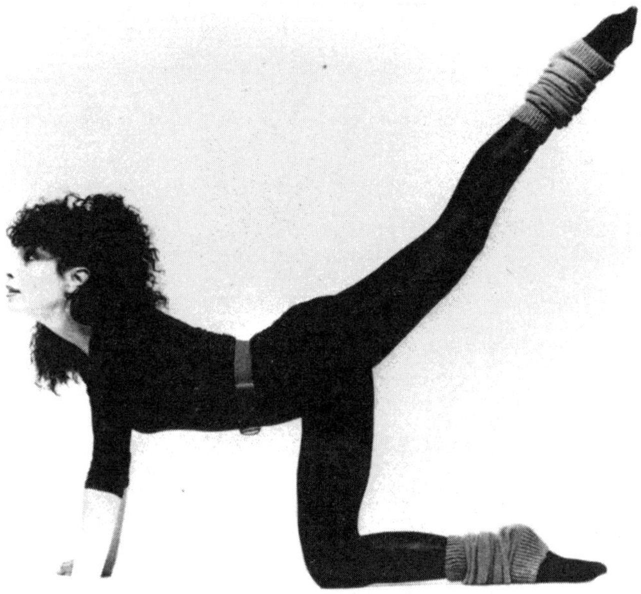

Lisa in the exercise studio.

In the 1980s, we opened an exercise studio and Lisa ran it. She had always been a dancer. She had a rockin' body. She taught aerobics and she was the most gorgeous woman I'd ever seen.

Then, all of a sudden, she wasn't feeling good. Tired all the time. No energy. She fought through it as best she could. We went to doctors. They thought she had multiple sclerosis.

I remember flying to Chicago during all of this. I was with Donna Mills and we were walking through O'Hare, and I saw this woman in a wheelchair. I was sure that would be my wife. My life. I was scared to death.

I was this dynamo, this whirlwind. All energy and no down time. How was this going to affect us? How was this going to affect me?

I've heard stories about men finding out that their wives had cancer. They couldn't deal with it and left. Or they cheated on them. I wouldn't do that to Lisa. I couldn't. She was—is—my soulmate, my best friend, my wife and my lover. She had stood with me through everything, and now this was my time to be with her.

When illness happens to a husband or wife, the other spouse has to dig deep and develop his or her own kind of strength. The one who's sick needs to know that the other is there for him or her. Their pain is so much worse than yours. Her pain was so much worse than mine.

I was scared.

I turned to bodybuilding. I didn't go out. I built a gym in the house. I worked out.

We went to more doctors. No one could diagnose her for sure. Maybe it was a brain tumor. Just migraines. Maybe she was an alcoholic. She had Lyme disease, lupus, arthritis. Nothing seemed right; no diagnosis made sense. Nothing was making her better.

She had had double-lumen breast implants shortly after we were married. Silicone inside of saline. Supposedly safe because if the silicone bled out it would bleed into the saline. A failproof situation. That's when she started to get sick. Finally, years later she was diagnosed with Chronic Fatigue Syndrome. There's no cure. There's just management.

The doctors never came right out and said that the implants had anything to do with it, though we knew—Lisa knew—instinctively that they did. Face it. Nothing you put into your body as a permanent fixture that wasn't there before can be good for you. It may make you look better, but the body doesn't want it. It rebels. It rebelled big time with Lisa.

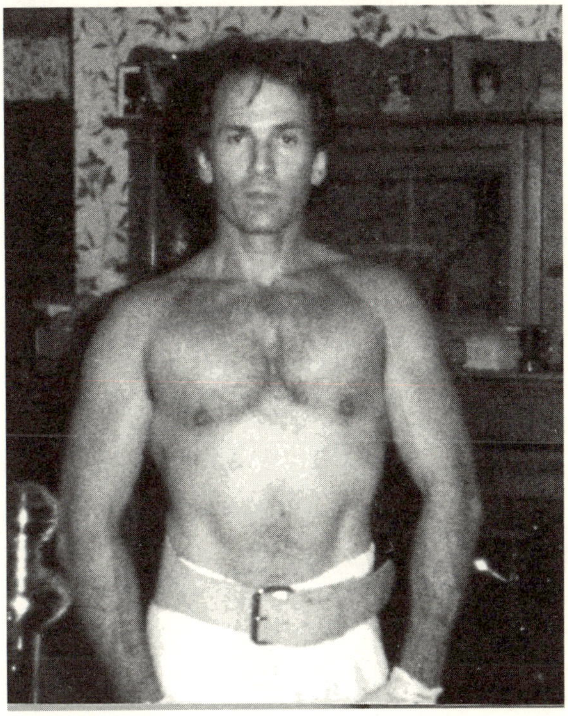

The incredible hulk at 40.

Tests eventually showed that the silicone from the implants had gotten into the cells in her body. Doctors ran a test called an antinuclear antibody test that detects unusual antibodies in the blood. These antinuclear antibodies are often found in people whose immune systems may be predisposed to cause inflammation against their own body tissues. The test looks for autoimmune diseases like systemic lupus, rheumatoid arthritis, Addison's disease, pernicious anemia, and pulmonary fibrosis. When Lisa was going through all of her tests, the inflammation present in her body, showing that cells were attacking their own nuclei, was sky high, hence the reason they thought she had arthritis or lupus. She didn't, and she finally had her implants removed. At my urging. Me, the guy who loves women and really loves breasts. I wanted them gone. They were making her sick.

Don't think the irony was lost on both of us.

One of the more ironic aspects of this whole ordeal was how hard it was to find a doctor who would actually remove the implants. We went to five, six, seven plastic surgeons (they're called cosmetic surgeons now) before we finally found Barbara Hayden. She did a different kind of surgery, using a method that didn't leave any scars. She actually did six hours of reconstruction. Lisa thought of her as an angel. I wasn't sure what to think. All I knew was that this woman helped my wife and helped our life. (Truth: If it wouldn't hurt her health, I would have her put the implants back in.)

When I look back on this now, it also seems that this is when everything started to go wrong. Lisa was sick (though getting better), the exercise studio was having trouble, partly because she was sick, and I was starting to lose friends to AIDS. The good life was starting to go bad.

As if to reinforce that, I lost one of my closest friends to the disease.

I had started out as a hairdresser back in the late 1960s. I was completely caught up in the *Shampoo* years of the 1970s, when every woman who came into my salon was fair game. I was a heterosexual hairdresser, which wasn't the norm. There's a reason the stereotype exists. I worked with a lot of hairdressers who were gay. I didn't really care. We were all professionals. I got very close to a number of these guys. One was Alan Clausen.

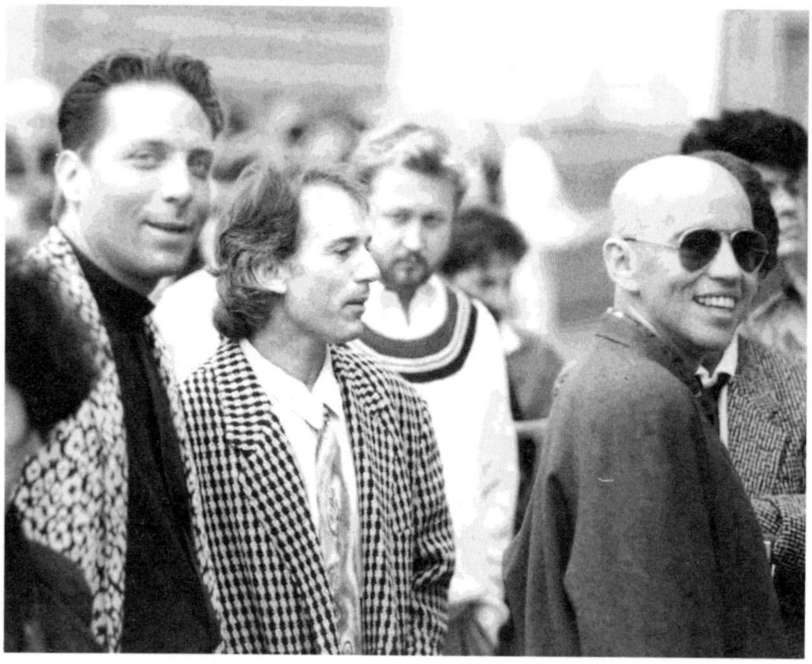

Me with Alan and Jose. Happy times.

Alan worked for Geri Cusenza when she opened her salon, Cassandra. You remember Geri. She stole all my hairdressers in the '70s. When Geri lost Cassandra, Alan came to work for me along with his partner, Jose Irizario. Paul hired them.

When Paul and I hired Alan, we did so for two reasons: we needed him to be a teacher, and I needed him to be part of my show team. We worked closely together for a long time. We also made Jose part of the show team, and the two of them traveled all over the country with me. It was Allen (me), Alan (him), Jose and a woman named Laurel (who was one of our partners who ran the new salon down in Newport Beach). We all had this incredible creative connection. We respected each other's work. No ego. That was something different. No egos between us. No "my cut's better than yours," "my style's bigger than yours."

Alan and I would travel and talk about guy things like cars and boats. He wasn't swishy or queeny. He didn't act gay around me. Whatever that even means. He had a chair in both my Beverly Hills salon and my Encino salon, and he was busy all the time.

Then, he stopped working. He just stopped. He didn't call in. Hell, he didn't call anyone. I asked around.

"He's sick," someone said.

Nothing prepared me for that.

"Sick?" *He's going to die.* I knew it then, knew that the plague had gotten him.

Evidently he was fighting every aspect of and for his life. He had broken up with Jose, got single for a while, then he married a woman (not a typo) who was quite a bit older than he was. We had traveled to London together once and he connected so much with Lisa that I almost got jealous. He "got" women like even a heterosexual stud like me never did.

It sucked.

One day, the phone rang. I answered and there was no one there. I was about to hang up. Suddenly, a raspy breath.

"Allen," came this ragged whisper that hurt my ears. I knew immediately that it was him.

"How are you, buddy?" I asked as I sat down, wishing that Lisa were there so I could hold her hand while talking to a dying man. But she was out. It was just me and the dog, who somehow sensed a change in my demeanor. He curled up at my feet while I held my head in my hand, the phone cradled on my shoulder.

"Well, you know, I've been better," he said, and I could tell he was trying to smile.

"Yeah," was all I could get out. I wanted to tell him I knew, tell him I missed him, tell him that he had become one of my closest friends, that I needed him. Instead I said "yeah." Master of the language.

"Listen," he said after a minute. I was listening. I AM LISTENING. I'm tied in knots here.

"I'm dying, Allen," he said. "Can you come?"

I got on my Harley and headed south, toward Laguna, a beautiful resort town along the coast, down in Orange County. There was a lot of money there—still is—four-star hotels, fancy cars, five-star restaurants. Alan had lived there for a little while.

I pulled up in front of his house. There were a couple of other cars, cars I didn't recognize. I didn't care. I had heard people talk about moving as if in a trance, as if some other force controlled their body. That's how I moved toward the front door. I can barely remember. I just know I made it up the front walkway and knocked at the door. Someone let me in. Alan was on the couch. He was very sick. I had never been around anyone who was dying before. I didn't know how to act. I went over to him and sat on the edge of the coffee table so I could talk to him.

I don't remember what we said.

I don't remember if I said good-bye.

He was dead a month later.

To this day, I think of Alan as a creative connection for me.

AIDS had come into my life, touching me personally. I can't say I only thought of Alan through all of this, though at the time, AIDS was still thought to be a largely gay disease. But it was a disease that you got by having sex. A disease that could kill you if you had sex. I had had a lot of sex. With a lot of women.

I'm not a religious person, but suddenly there was a disease that slammed the door shut on the wildest sexual time since the Roman Empire. It stopped the hetero world dead in its tracks. Everyone was totally paranoid.

You had to wonder what the hell God was thinking.

After the shock of Alan's death, the reality set in. I was worried. During my single days, there were some lonely nights where I was with the totally wrong kind of girl. By wrong kind of girl I mean this: Sometimes, some girls had sex with gay men, just for fun.

I had a test. It was negative.

But I'd lost one of my best friends, and my wife was still sick. The body studio was losing money, the salons were doing well, but my partnership with Paul Canter was showing some strains.

Things had been so good, so easy, for so long. I had a feeling that things were going to change.

Soon.

seven

The Sounds of War and Loss

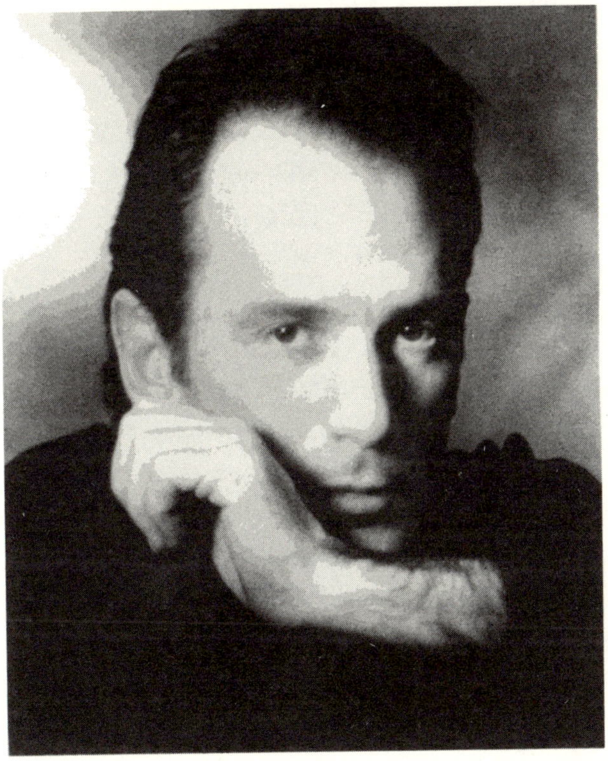

When I was doing shows, traveling around the country, I was incredibly happy. Every show I did had a theme, like "Follow the Yellow Brick Road to Your Future as a Hairdresser." I was doing shows for KMS, which I produced, directed and put together. I created a method of working. I had people from all over coming to these shows. I saw a Japanese team once, and they were moving their shears so fast, it was like they were carving meat. It was like being at a Tappan grill. I had to do that; that was my missing link. When they finished and started styling, they lost it. But the shears were amazing. All 7" of them. I polished those shears like Ginsu knives so they sparkled in the light. I loved the Japanese and they loved me.

I practiced. And practiced. And practiced. With 7-inch shears I practiced until I got faster and faster so that when I was on stage, it would be pure energy, pure fun. I wanted to blow people away. We were all connected, the models, the hair stylists, the shears, the dry ice. I remember this one piece, from Yellow Brick Road. The song was "Ease on Down the Road" and I had ten hairdressers on stage at one time, cutting and styling hair. There was a yellow brick road on stage and we were definitely easing down it. It was amazing.

With KMS, I also started including comedy in my shows. Suddenly I was a stand-up. I could control the audience with laughter and stories of celebrities. Once I had them laughing I could do and say anything I wanted. I talked, I preached, I motivated, I taught, and I was a great hairdresser who did great work.

No ego. (Honest.)

I went to Atlantic City and did a show, taking the stage before the Paul Mitchell team. Mel Joseph, from Clairol, was in the audience. He saw my rock show and couldn't believe it. He'd never seen that kind of energy. He convinced me to take the place of the Chadwicks (John and Suzanne), who were working for Clairol at the time and eventually went to Mitchell. I said sure.

The Chadwicks were the first hairdressers I'd seen perform in a show on stage, in New York. I thought their way of teaching was amazing. John was a bit stuffy, but Suzanne was adorable. Suzanne and I had a creative connection, even without knowing each other. I think she had the hots for me. Of course, I think everyone has the hots for me.

When I took their place, John wasn't thrilled. Can't imagine why.

I was young, not at all corporate. A little bit of a wild card. I was the only hairdresser at the time to say "fuck" on stage. But I used it in a way that made complete sense. Really.

The F-bomb stimulates an audience of hairdressers like nothing else. Anytime you go to a comedy show, the F-bomb gets a laugh. A rise. I would ask the audience, "Wouldn't you like to say, if you don't want to do what I want, then get the fuck out of my chair?"

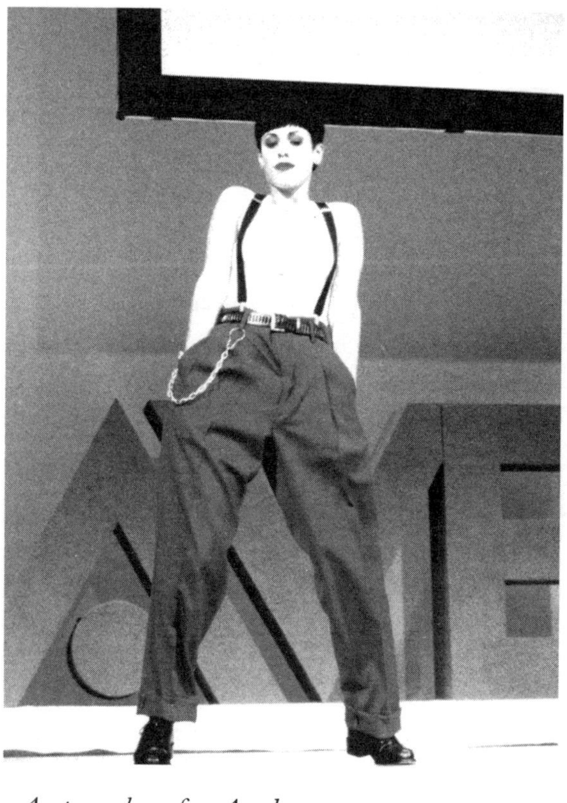

A stage show for Aveda.

And they'd go crazy. Because it's not how we EVER talk to clients. It's a release because a lot of stylists have trouble telling a client how they feel, what they want to do creatively, so they become the client's dog. Tease it, make it bigger. The hairdresser does it, but doesn't love it. They're working to make the clients happy, and it has to be more than that. I tapped into their fantasies of what they always wanted.

Suddenly I found myself in New York City at Studio 54, for Mel and Clairol, which in the 1980s was the place to be. We were doing a show. Had a huge turnout of hairdressers. The model call? No one really had the hair texture we needed to create a specific look, and not one of them wanted her hair cut. And not one of them was under 200 pounds. The spandex just wasn't working for this crowd. I flipped out. I had a show in mind and I was going to produce what I wanted. But I was ranting about the model call.

"Allen," said a timid assistant.

"WHAT?" I barked.

"We have one," she said.

"One?" I shouted. "We have one freakin' model? Christ! Where is she?"

She walks out. Struts, really. At 2 feet tall and close to 500 pounds. A slight embellishment.

"No," I said calmly.

"But—"

"NO! NO! NO!" I was trying to remain calm, though it clearly wasn't working. "Go out onto the streets and find me some fucking models. Now!"

My team scattered out onto the streets of New York. They approached all kinds of girls, offering them $50 to come on stage and get their hair cut. My team should have been doing hair. But they were looking for models.

We found two.

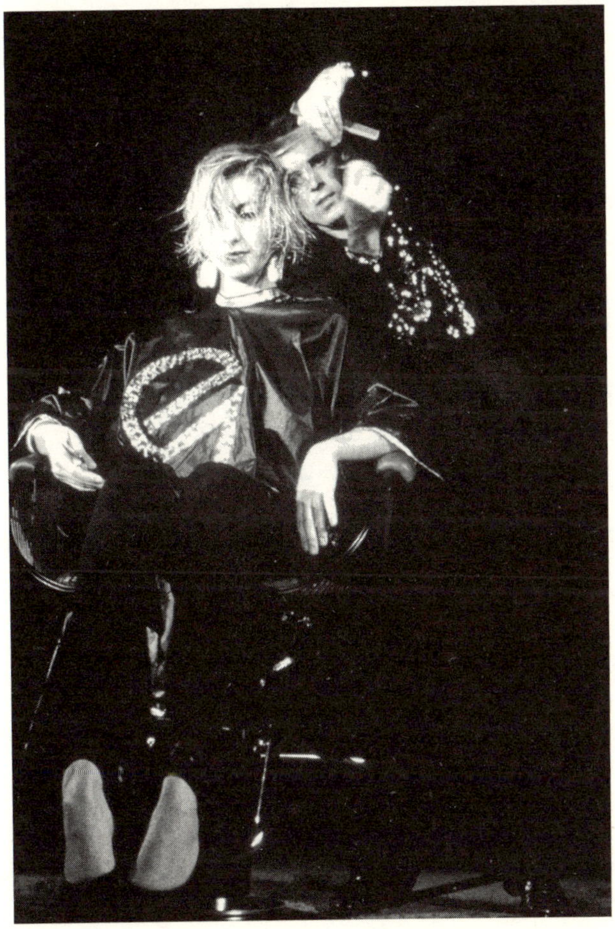

Me on stage, cutting hair to music.

Two.

TWO!

I called a guy at a model agency.

"You g-g-g-g-got-ta help me. I'm fre-fre-fre-freakin' out he-he-he-here."

Two hours later, just before we took the stage, in walked ten models from the agency. The most gorgeous girls I'd ever seen.

Clairol had set up an open bar. Something I'd always asked for there NOT to be. Ninety percent of the hairdressers were from Queens or Long Island, and in their wildest dreams they couldn't have imagined getting into Studio 54. They were partying and drinking, and I. Was. Furious. I insulted a couple of people. It wasn't my best show.

I loved Clairol. They paid me $10,000 per show. I was the highest paid platform artist in the world. I flew first class. I had limousine transfers. It was the most exciting time of my life.

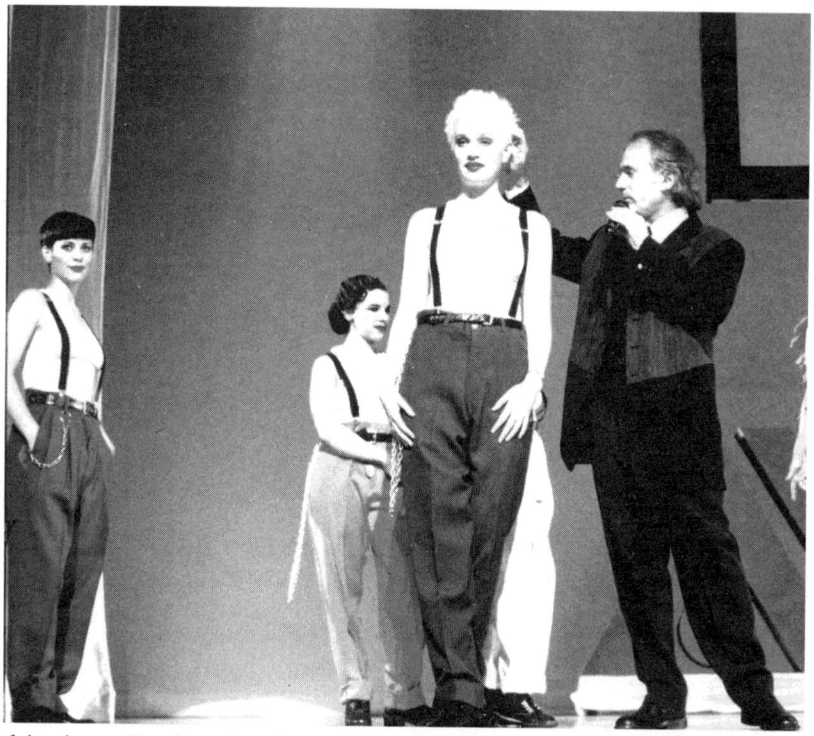

During this time, Paul and I decided to convince Mel Joseph to leave Clairol, come with us and run our new product company, to be president of a little thing we decided to do called "CarboSilk." It was carbohydrates and silk proteins for hair. Because of all the bodybuilding I was doing, because Lisa was sick and I was working out all the time, I was consumed with carbohydrates. I wanted to capitalize on the carbohydrate phase. I figured that doing it for hair was the best of all worlds.

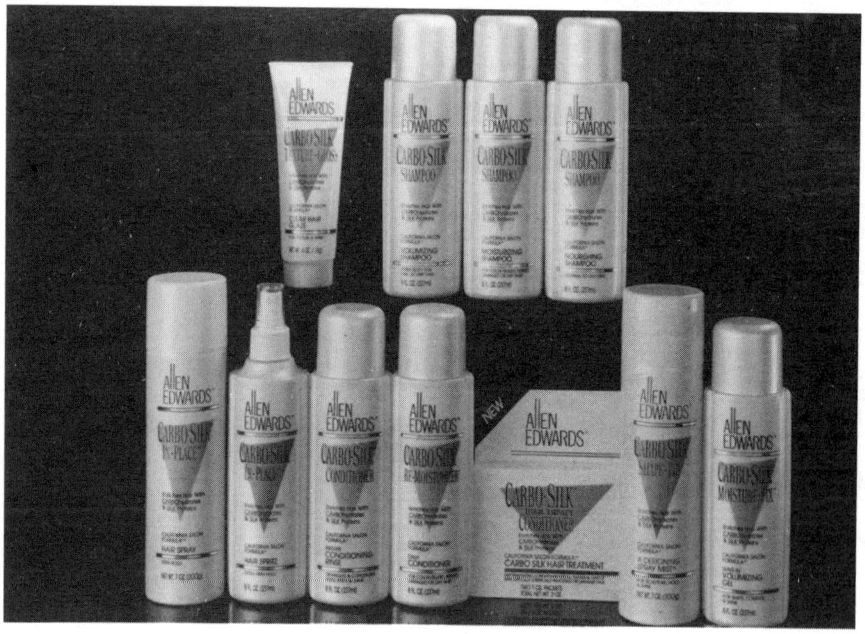

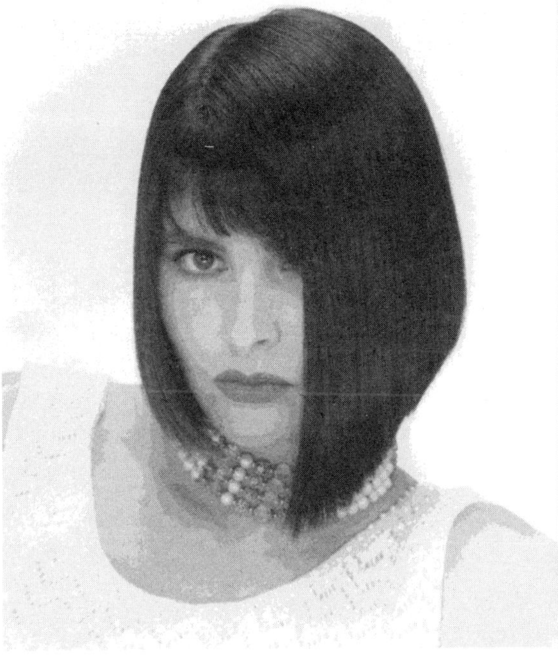

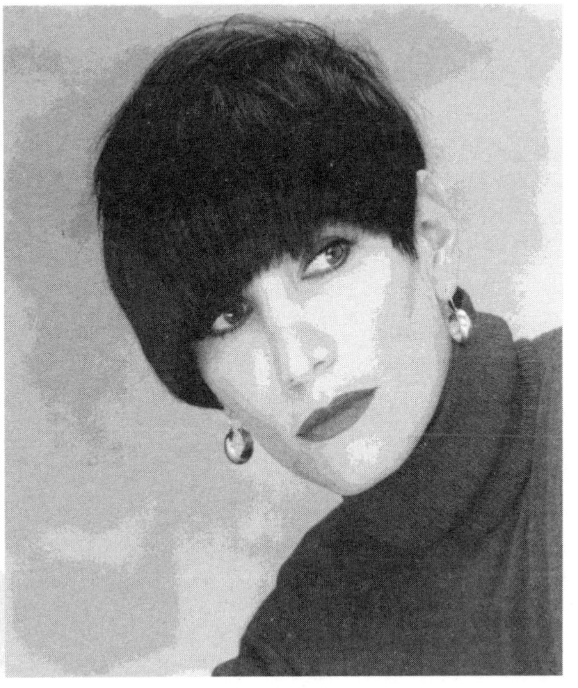

Styles created with CarboSilk.

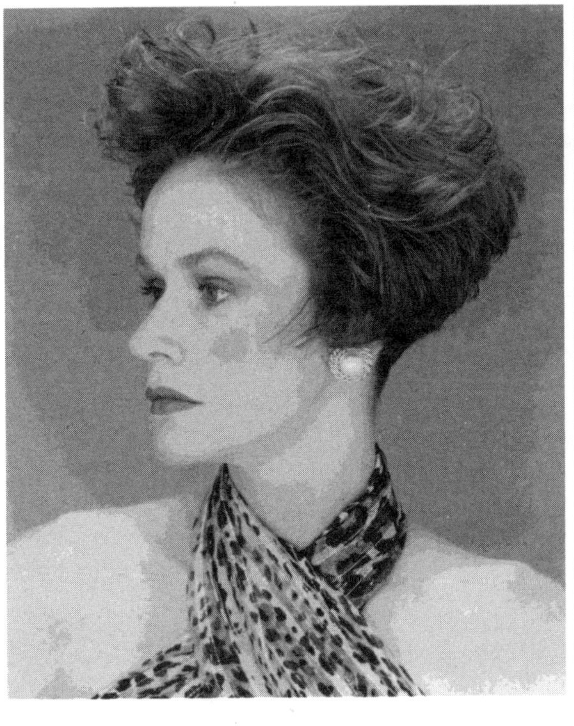

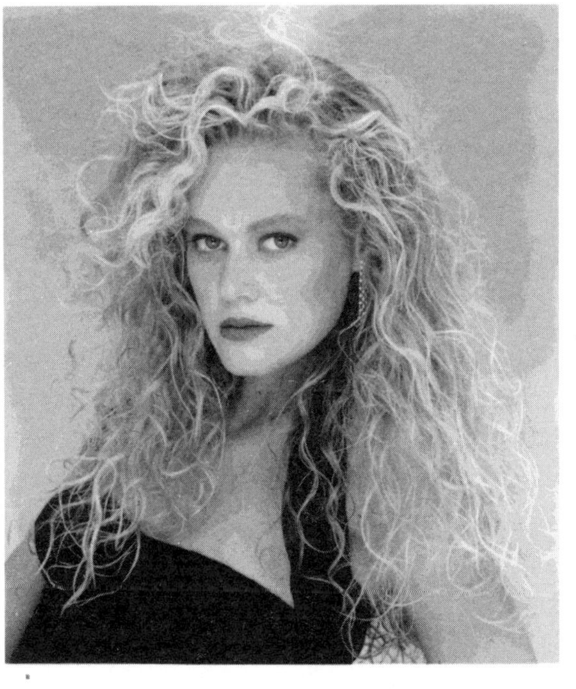

Mel came to Los Angeles and we had this big meeting. Paul, however, decided that HE wanted to be the president of the company. He had no idea how to run a hair products company. That's why we wanted Mel. Mel was brilliant when it came to running a product company and had all the connections.

Mel took it all in and sat back in his chair and smiled. "I left Clairol to be… vice president?"

He had this look on his face that pegged us completely as amateurs. He was right.

We made the product, but we had a hard time getting it off the ground. Mel had all these distributor connections, and they weren't buying it. He was pissed and stuck in the role of VP, and didn't want to work under Paul.

In the middle of one meeting, Paul decided that the company should lease him a car. I went nuts.

"How can you even think about getting a car when we're not making any money?"

It was the beginning of the end.

With CarboSilk, Paul wanted to bring in a thousand partners to help us. Mel was setting up shows to pitch the product. We were going to be in Chicago, Boston, Miami. I'd work all day in the salon, cutting hair, then take the red-eye back East to do these shows. We started selling some product, but we were running out of money. Mel and Paul were fighting. It was a nightmare.

We all sat around one night, with a bottle of brandy, asking each other what the hell we were going to do with the company.

Trevor Sorbie and Irvin Rusk were up and coming. Ogie started pulling distributors from us because they ran on bullshit. They got magazines to do write-ups on them. It was all hype. They had no team, no education.

Sebastian started advertising in *Vogue* and *Bazaar.* And we were dying on the vine. But we owed $300,000, $100,000 of it mine, and my house was tied up in the money. If we went bankrupt, which Ogie eventually did, I'd lose. We'd all lose.

"What the hell are we going to do?" I asked. I knew I sounded like I'd just lost my dog.

The next day, Paula Kent Meehan from Redken called. She was interested in buying the company, I thought, and wanted to know if I could come and meet with her.

The day of the meeting, I had the worst case of the flu I'd ever had in my life. I looked and felt like death. Yet another metaphor for everything that was starting to rain down on me. I sat in on this meeting with Paula and all of her people. And I had to make a decision. Because they didn't want to buy CarboSilk; they wanted to bankrupt it and take me into another company. I wanted the money to pay back the second and third mortgage I'd taken out on my house. Paula had already been screwed by another guy, so she wouldn't give me a dime.

All I could think while I was sitting there, looking around at this corporate office, was "This is not what I want to do." The room had this big, dark, wood table, with fingerprints left every time someone put his or her hand down. Black swivel chairs. It was archaic. The people sitting in the black swivel chairs were all old, too. Paula was at her end. It was like the Mafia. It made Clairol look like the hippest company on the planet. I didn't want to be hooked up with a company that was full of cobwebs.

The whole thing wasn't doing it for me.

They were talking about me like I wasn't in the room. Which, truth be told, was sort of correct since I had faded a bit into the paneling because I felt so crappy.

"We could go retail," someone suggested.

"Allen Edwards retail? I don't see it," someone else countered.

"We could take him OTC or into a beauty supply."

No one wanted to commit to anything.

I'M SITTING RIGHT HERE, I wanted to shout. And I'm not going over the counter. And I may be pulling an Exorcist here if you people don't shut the hell up.

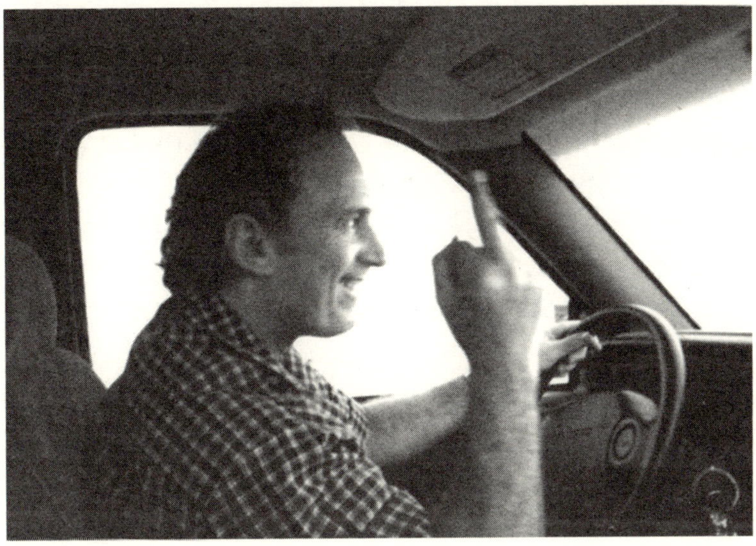

'Nuf said.

After hours with no progress, the meeting broke up and I went home, sick as a dog. I got a call from a guy named Jack Forsolino (he liked to be called The Force. How's that for ego?). Same day, no kidding. His wife Beth had been one of the producers on the Vidal Sassoon show. I had been a guest and she really liked me. Jack was this huge guy, like 400 pounds, very Italian. He wanted to buy the company and take it retail.

I met with him several days later, after my flu had flown, and we drove through Little Italy with wives in tow and Lisa asked, quietly, in case the answer was yes: "Is this connected to the mob?"

Jack laughed, this big 400-pound laugh, and he bellowed out "No!" Almost broke the car windows.

And of course, I believed him because I'd have believed anything right then. Never mind the fact that he was pointing things out like:

"That spot, right there? That's where they got Lucky Luciano. You can still see the blood if you look hard."

I'd become a bit player on *The Sopranos.* I was the guest star who didn't even get a whole name because the guy was going to be toast by the end of the first act.

But Jack, he wanted to buy the company. Bada bing!

"I'll give you $400,000 right now, and I've got $3 mil to take it retail."

Sounded good to me. I owned a big piece of the company. I'd sell to Jack, not Paula and Redken.

I felt like I was being wined and dined. Like a girl at the prom. Who wanted to dance the most with Allen?

Unfortunately, I was about to be stood up. Left at the altar. Dismissed.

Jack decided to remake the product. He was running the company now, running CarboSilk, so there wasn't anything any of us could do. He wanted to take a $3 million life insurance policy out on me. That way, if they didn't make any money on the product, and I disappeared, they'd still make money. (Bada bing.)

It made me a little nervous. I could see my life flashing before my eyes. Brake lines cut on the Ferrari, a salon blowing up after an aerosol can ignited mysteriously, a pair of shears shoved into my carotid artery.

Luckily for me, the insurance company thought the same thing. They didn't bite.

Jack started to get a little panicky after that. He started trying to buy his way into all the markets. I had this PR person and he wanted her to call the editor of *Los Angeles Magazine* and bribe him with a Rolex watch to put me on the cover.

"Who do you think you are? Al Capone?" she asked, sort of as a joke. Sort of not.

He really did think he was Capone.

Time went on. He kept telling me how great everything was going, but then he started running out of money. He ran right into the late 1980s recession. He was broke. As a last resort, he hired a distributor, and the distributor and I went to the corporate offices of Target to try to sell the idea of CarboSilk. The guy looked at our concept. He liked the way it looked, loved the way it smelled.

"How you gonna sell it?" he asked.

"We've got a $6 million budget," the distributor said. With a straight face. While I'm having a meltdown across the table. Internally, though, so no one could see it. Because we had about a six cent budget.

Still, Target took the line and put it in six stores.

Didn't sell a thing.

In six months, it was out of Target, the CarboSilk company went bankrupt, and my retail experience was over. I was still standing behind the chair, still cutting hair. I felt like crap. All I could think about was how it had all started.

Jon.

Jon Peters was the first one who trained hairdressers. He was the first to have an assistant. Teaching people how to do hair made them more loyal employees. It was better than hiring from the outside. It was a practice I subscribed to then. A practice I still subscribe to.

In my salons, my hairdressers were getting busier and busier, but like any business, everyone always wanted to go further and make more money. In my mind, you have to deserve it. You have to be loyal; you have to be a team player. And the business has to keep growing. There are always ways of compensating and helping people out.

In the 1980s, the times were definitely changing. There was a big salon that opened up in Beverly Hills. About 10,000 square feet. Who the owner was isn't important. But he had to fill that space, so he started going after hairdressers, offering them God-knows what to get them to leave where they were.

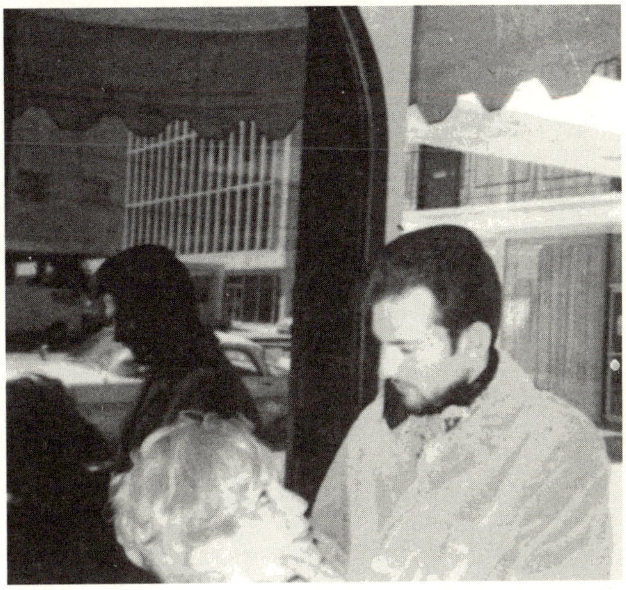

Me in the salon, 20 years old.

For me, it was never about the money. It was about working for the best name, the best salon, the one that could teach me the most.

But that wasn't what this guy believed. When you have a competitor who starts giving it away, it makes it difficult to compete. Owners don't always play on the same playing field. Sometimes they rig the game.

This is how the war started.

The Hairdresser Wars

I never had a problem with people leaving my salons because they were going to do shows all over the country. Good for them. Hell, I did that myself, as often as I could. That was life and I was motivated, too. People leaving my salons to go to a desperate owner who was giving it away was chicken shit. I would train them, build them, mentor them, and they'd leave.

Some hairdressers only wanted the money. For me, it was always the art, always about getting better.

I call it the hairdresser's mentality. It's artistic, a little bit flaky, with the constant need of a babysitter. If hairdressers leave and go to another salon, they lose clients. But they should lose clients. They don't have the drive and the dedication; they don't have the focus. They're in it for 9 to 5. And they can make decent money. Not necessarily great money. Not $100,000 a year. That's tough. But they also don't have the pressure of working in a corporate environment, where it's easy to get canned. Hairdressers don't get canned very easily.

One of the reasons I never quit cutting hair is because it gives me the security to keep going even if something bad happens. In the '80s, there was bad happening. We

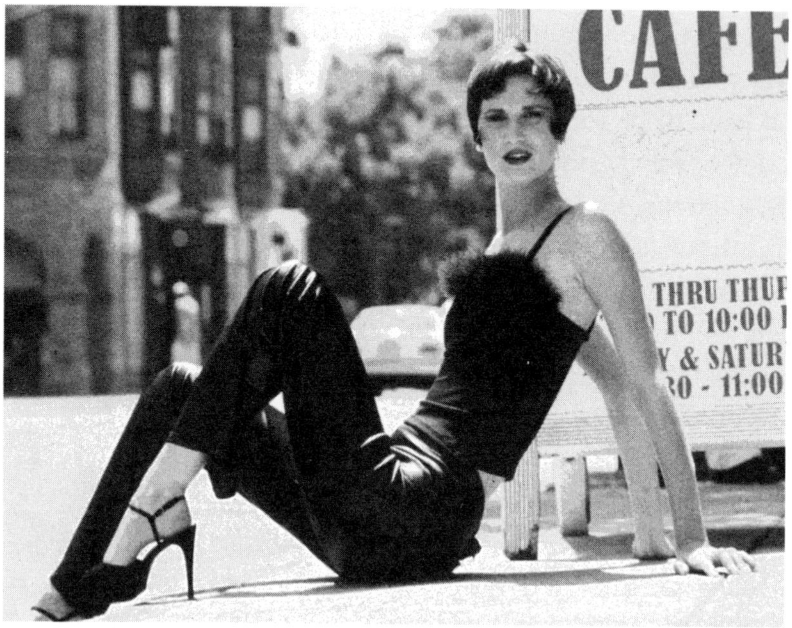

It was always the art, always about getting better.

tried to come up with creative ways to pay people who had been with us for a long time. Sometimes it worked…

This one day, Paul says to me, "We just lost three facialists."

"Three?"

"Three," he confirmed. "Once came to me crying and complaining about nothing even worth repeating. She quit. Then the one she was complaining about quit."

"And the third?" I asked, rubbing my eyes.

"I fired her because she was pissing me off."

Sometimes it didn't work at all.

It was like the woman who had been making $2,000 a week and I couldn't get her to settle down. She was all over the place, disrupting the whole salon. I finally had to fire her as well, and suddenly she was bad-mouthing me all over town. I was the bad guy because I was the boss; I was the businessman. When people leave you, as the owner, you will always be the bad guy. I don't like that, even though I understand it.

Worse, the clients blamed me. I felt like I was starting to fight a losing battle. What had been fun in the '70s and early '80s was slowly becoming torture. I still loved doing hair, but the business side was killing me.

Paul

With Paul, my first partner, I was really making some serious money and becoming famous at the same time. I was always the one in the limelight because I had to be. It

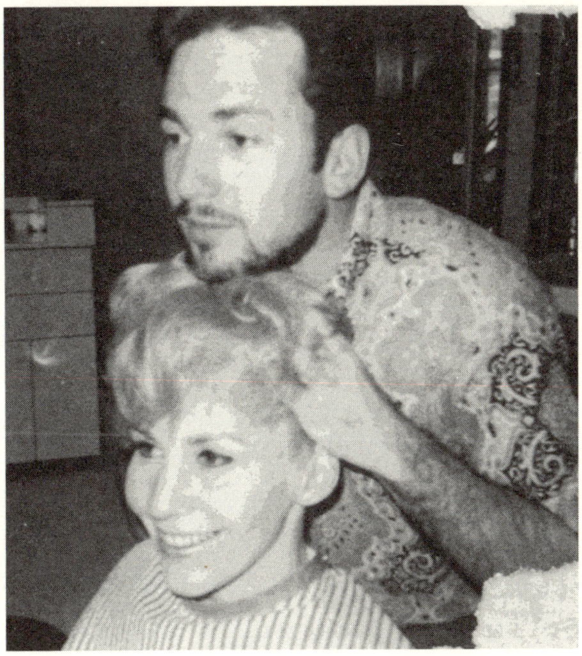
Me, still in the salon, loving it.

started when I was a kid playing trumpet, only now the instrument was my shears in my hands.

For a long time, Paul and I were equals because we were both cutting hair, both seeing a ridiculous amount of clients. We'd split the profits. It was a perfect partnership. We were both feeding the business and feeding our wallets.

Then…

"I think I'm going to stop doing hair," Paul said to me one afternoon in Encino. "Concentrate on the business of the business."

"The business of the business is hair," I pointed out, rightly, I thought.

"You know what I mean," he said. "I mean, you're the one people know. You're practically a rock star. You're the draw. Hell, it's your name on the door."

I couldn't argue with that. I WAS the one who did the shows. It WAS my name on the door. Did that mean it was also MY money in HIS pocket? I'd never looked at it that way before, but as soon as he stopped cutting hair, I started to.

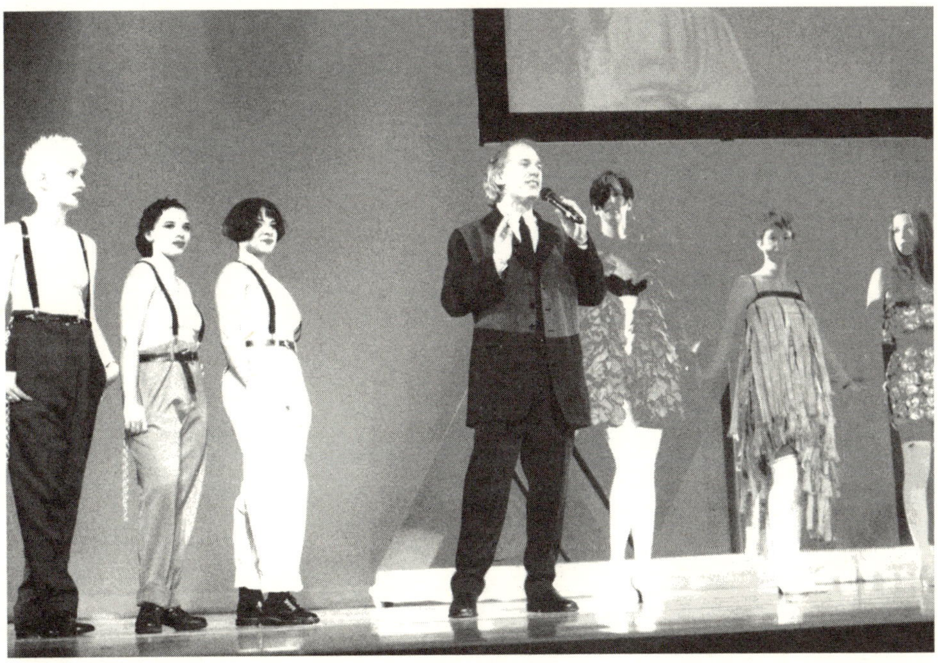

Paul and I had always had this amazing relationship. We understood each other; we complemented each other. He wanted to be behind the scenes and I wanted to be out front, stirring up trouble and getting publicity. I was the de facto expert, doing TV, being the performer. He'd already been taking care of a lot of the business side, and I thought he was good at it. It had been a perfect formula. Two hairdressers in business together. He kept what he made, I kept what I made, and then we split the profits. Perfect.

Yeah, right.

When he quit doing hair, he quit completely. I guess I thought he meant he was going to start cutting back on how much hair he was doing. I guess I should have paid more attention to the "stop doing hair" part. He also gave himself a salary, which ended up basically being the profit because he was no longer bringing in clients. He wasn't keeping what he made because he wasn't making anything. The salon was. I didn't get any of the profit anymore because it all went to pay him.

We had been partners for more than 20 years. I believed in him. He had convinced me that he was going to do better for us by just running the business side and not standing behind the chair anymore, and I was so busy being the star that I ended up falling to earth. I ended up getting screwed.

I felt like I was producing all the income and he was keeping it. I was so frustrated and stressed, even more than usual. I went to an astrologer (I know, I know. It seemed like a good idea at the time. Even Nancy Reagan was doing it) and he was supposedly pretty reputable. A lot of celebrities were going to him to find out if they should do a particular movie. I figured I had nothing to lose.

I walked into the guy's office. I don't know what I expected, but there were no black velvet curtains, no talismans hanging from the ceiling. Hell, there wasn't even a crystal ball. We sat on the couch. I felt like I was in therapy.

"So tell me," he said very seriously as he was gazing deeply into my eyes. I rolled mine. He smiled. "It's OK," he said. "Just relax."

Like I said, therapy.

But I told him what was going on with Paul and how I felt like I was being screwed and that I didn't know what to do.

He took my hand. I took it back. He took it again.

"Allen," he said quietly.

"Wh-wh-what?" I asked, equally quietly. Damned stutter showed itself at the most awkward times.

"It's already happening."

"What's already happening?" I asked.

"The end of your partnership."

"And how do you know this?" I asked.

"Because your stars are aligned," he said with confidence.

"Aligned with what?" I asked.

"With the universe. With you. They're pointing you in a particular direction. You're already going there. You're just not believing it because you're not sure you're ready. But if you allow the stars to lead you, you'll find what you seek," he said by way of explanation.

I was confused.

"What?"

"You'll find what you seek," he said again.

"But I don't know what I seek. I was ho-ho-hoping you'd tell me."

"But I just did."

"You see the end of my partnership with Paul," I said, finally getting it. And he nodded.

I drove back to the salon, thinking about everything that had transpired, not just with the astrologer, but also over the course of the last few months. We'd lost the CarboSilk business. We were losing money in the salons.

I thought about how being a partner is harder than being married. In a partnership, you have to have communication. You have to have emotion. We could scream and yell at each other and then hug and make up. And you have to do all of that without the sex.

A Little Sidebar about Partners

I've probably had more partners than any hairdresser in the country. The big question: why?

What was lacking in me that I felt I always needed to have a partner? For me, partners gave more security and strength; it was someone to throw things off of. Two people working together can be very powerful. But each partner should know his place; know what he does best and excel in that.

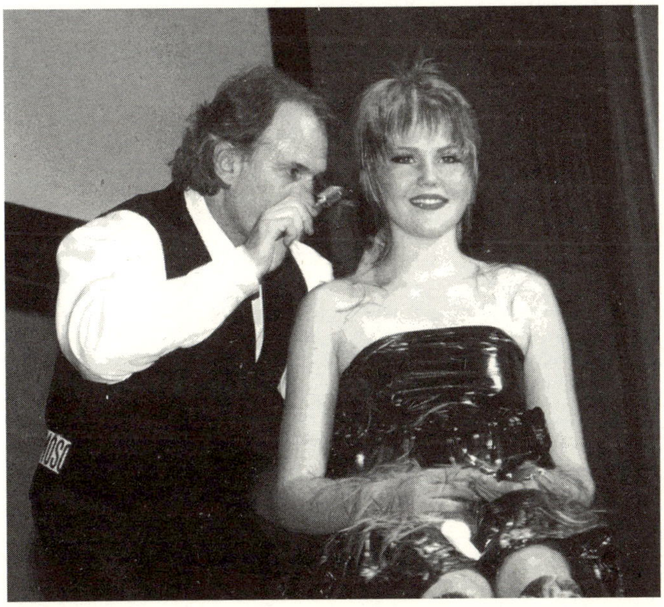

On stage.

What I do best is cut hair, do shows, bring in PR. I'll work harder than anyone else I know, longer hours, and make us all a lot of money. What I do worst? I'm very unorganized, and only anal when I have to be. I hate paperwork, and I hate doing things I don't like.

My first partners were Jon Peters and Paul Canter. Jon wasn't a good partner because it was all about Jon. Paul was a good partner for a while. He knew what he did well, which was negotiating, schmoozing, and getting front row seats in Las Vegas. Paul knew how to excel in what I do best. He was a great man, behind the scenes. He never had a big ego and never wanted to be me. Our partnership lasted 20 years.

I had other partners, like Frank and Laurel. She was a great hairdresser who motivated people. Frank was a great businessman. We all communicated well, and most of all, we knew how to party. That partnership lasted 15 years or so, during the same time as Paul.

Richard Olette was a short-term affair. Loved having me as a partner but didn't like sharing the limelight. He was a great businessman, probably one of the best of all of them, and he had a hard time sharing. We were only partners for two or three years.

Claudio Lazo was a great partner for the first three years. But he didn't really get the idea of making money off of the Allen Edwards name. He was probably better off on his own, which he is now. We were partners for ten years.

I always knew where my weaknesses were and was always looking for someone to fill in the missing pieces. I was smart enough to bring in someone to complement me. They did the management that I couldn't and didn't want to do. Ultimately that made us a stronger team. Because I know what I do well, and I know what I don't do well.

My very best partner is Lisa, who runs the business side of the business today. Not just because she's my wife and she's the only one I can mess around with without being sued, but she does everything that I hate to do. She's organized, anal, and anybody who's reading this book should steal her away from me to run their business.

Bottom line: When you want a partner, don't partner with someone who does the same thing that you do. You need someone who complements you, not someone who mirrors you.

Lesson: Think twice when choosing a partner.

Back to Paul

Paul and I had made a lot of money together for a long time. We made it largely because of my name, which was fine with him. He didn't have an ego. In a sense, he was Allen Edwards with me, always behind me, always supportive of me and any crazy idea I might come up with.

We had had so much fun together, making money, spending money, screwing our brains out (in the 1970s). I knew he rationalized taking the profit because I was out front, getting all the accolades. And he was a great idea guy. He knew how to use my name to make money. When we lost those 27 people to Geri Cusenza when she opened Cassandra, he knew how to rebuild the salon by touting the name. Come to Allen Edwards. Work at Allen Edwards.

Allen Edwards rocks.

But it seemed like his life was falling apart behind the scenes. It was affecting his decision-making skills. His brother-in-law became our accountant. It seemed calculating to me. Not that he was stealing from me, or cooking the books. Not really. But something wasn't right about the whole thing, and I wondered what was taking Paul in the wrong direction. He played the stock market, but that wasn't it. I noticed that Saturdays, the busiest day of the week in the salon, he would go play golf. Even if he'd only done hair on Saturdays, he could have made $1000 and we would have been better off. He could have done it all differently.

But he didn't.

I ended the partnership and bought him out. It was 1985. He got the salon in Encino: Allen Edwards Encino. (It's still called Allen Edwards Encino. Paul is still running it.) But I gave up my name. Not a smart move when your name is your entire reputation.

From there it was a downward spiral of ending relationships and bad money decisions. Lisa and I closed the body studio. It was losing money.

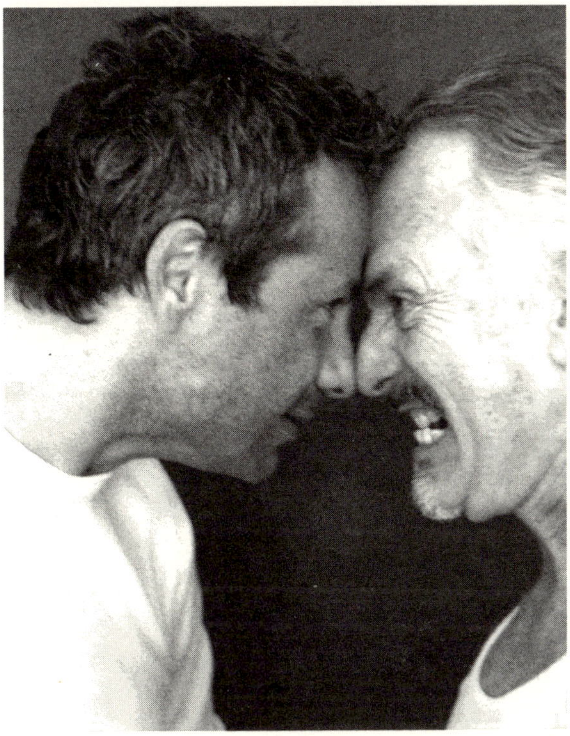

Partners. The beginning of the end.

I took on another partner in my Studio City salon. The problem with being my partner is that you have to understand that you will never be Allen Edwards. You don't necessarily get to go on TV, and you don't necessarily get the PR. I don't think some of my partners ever really understood that. They were all fine in the beginning until their egos got in the way. But if they opened their eyes to see that all the publicity I bring is also building the salon, we'd all be better off. The name, if not the man, gets PR, and PR gets clients, and clients fill the salon.

And I get to do what I do best, which is perform and build the name.

I had a salon in Newport Beach as well, with Laurel and Frank Chirico as partners. They were like family to me, and Laurel, in a lot of ways, was like a second wife. We traveled together, we did shows together. She was one of the most creative people I've ever worked with, to this day. They actually helped me to buy out Paul, but the dynamic between all of us was changing. They were getting very involved with Toni & Guy, and I was getting involved with Aveda. We were coming from different places, but it was working, or at least I thought it was. Sort of.

When I bought out Paul, I put together yet another business relationship (though not a partnership) with a guy named Richard Olette. Laurel hated him, but I thought he was OK. Richard and I were going to do less expensive salons together, in shopping malls. He even thought we could go into outlet malls. We weren't going to call them Allen Edwards. They were going to be Colors, Cuts and Perms by Allen Edwards. He licensed my name to use in three salons, sort of as a trial run.

My ego said, "Fuck yeah." My partners screamed, "You're out of your fucking mind." I hadn't talked to Laurel and Frank about it. I just did it. Laurel went berserk, accusing me of betraying them, of betraying their trust, of undermining the business, of cheapening my name, of taking chances with other people's lives, of the Kennedy assassination. She was right about everything (except the Kennedy thing). I shouldn't have done it. I had descended into this strange place somehow, and I was hurting everyone around me. Especially me.

The salon started emptying out. Frank bought a boat. They put together a deal with T & G and left me in the dust.

Well, that's not entirely true. I had Richard. And I still had Woodland Hills, Studio City and Beverly Hills.

Bada bing.

eight

Losing Beverly Hills

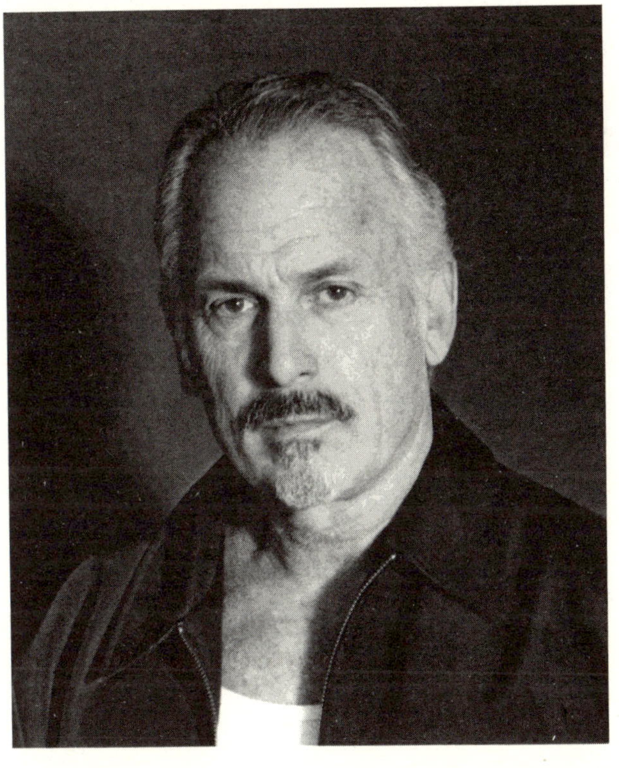

I was playing a serious game of virtual Monopoly with everyone, and I was losing all my holdings, all my hotels, all my money. I had a get-out-of-jail-free card and a go-directly-to-jail, do-not-pass-go, do-not-collect-$200 card. I just wasn't sure which one would be used.

Richard Olette put my name on his existing salon in Santa Ana. Problem: it was a little too close to the Newport Beach Allen Edwards salon, and Laurel came unglued.

"How can you do that?" she screamed at me. "You're bastardizing our business, bastardizing your own name! Who does that? What is wrong with you?"

The thing is, I didn't see anything wrong with what I was doing. It didn't seem like competition to me. Yes, both salons carried my name, but each catered to a different clientele. One was like Spago; one was like Wolfgang Puck Café.

So there we were, with a salon in the Santa Ana mall, seven miles from Allen Edwards Newport Beach, another in Irvine and another soon to be open in San Diego. Laurel and Frank absolutely hated Richard, hated the fact that I had these other lower-end salons. Gradually, Allen Edwards Newport Beach lost all of its hairdressers. And I lost two more partners when Laurel and Frank decided to buy me out.

Fine, I thought. So what that we'd been together for a long time? So what that they didn't like what I was doing? So fucking what? They don't need me, I don't need them. The problem with that kind of thinking is that you do need people. You also need to let them know what's going on. That was my mistake, though I still don't think it was a wrong decision.

Within months both Laurel and Frank were with Toni & Guy. They still are. Looking back, I would have done it differently. I handled it all very badly. Hell, I would have done exactly what they did if I'd been thinking more clearly.

But I was thinking like Allen.

My deal with Richard was getting trickier all the time. Licensing is a very weird business. People expect too much. When Richard and I opened a salon in Ontario Mills, I went on television, not necessarily to promote it, but just to promote, well, me, and suddenly we had 300 clients. But we didn't have enough hairdressers, didn't have enough education, so those clients got mad. They thought they were getting Allen Edwards. They weren't. They were just getting my name on the door.

Richard was a better businessman than me, but he really had a big ego. He didn't like his hairdressers looking up to me. He had been in the salon industry for years and had two other salons that were grossing more than $1 million a year. He decided to open a salon in San Diego, but I had just opened Brentwood and he didn't think I was paying enough attention to San Diego. Not true. I traveled back and forth constantly. The problem was that he had put the San Diego salon on the first floor of a mall, near the movie theaters. Everyone goes to the movies; it seemed like a great place to put a salon. The problem was that the theater wasn't open yet, so the salon wasn't getting much walk-by traffic.

Then Richard decided not to pay me royalties. I was mad. I was going to get even.

I managed to light him on fire and ruin our relationship when I told him his wife had him by the balls, and that he should start controlling her instead of just letting her control him. I wasn't sure that it was true, but I was really pissed off about him not paying me royalties. He was wrong. We both knew he was wrong. And after my lawyer got ahold of him, that wrong was corrected.

That was the end of that.

Tokyo, Japan: Remembered

OK, fine. Things had fallen apart in the U.S. I had lost Encino to Paul, I had lost Newport Beach to Laurel and Frank. I had lost my little foray into licensing to Richard. I had lost my product line to Jack.

But I still had my memories of Tokyo. For some reason, all of this loss made me nostalgic for Tokyo. They loved me in Tokyo.

When I had gone there years before, I had licensed another franchise salon called Taya Salon, and actually made some money. This was in the 1980s, when the Japanese loved all things American. The louder and more flamboyant, the better. Now, I was never flamboyant (other than my decorating), but I could definitely be loud. My stage shows were legendary, not just for the music but for the talking, shouting, and fun.

In Tokyo, the man who franchised my name (the name again) wanted a Beverly Hills feel for visiting tourists and Americans living in Japan. He hired hairdressers from all over and franchised my name for seven years.

After seven years, he decided it wasn't going to work. He had opened other salons, took them onto the Tokyo stock exchange and made a fortune.

That was that.

God, how I loved Japan.

My first experience there was with a company called Lux. J. Walter Thompson, who was doing a commercial for Lux, knew me from SunSilk. They called me to help. Evidently, the hair was a disaster. I went down, told them what they were doing wrong. That was that.

Or so I thought.

They ended up sending me to Japan for a day to do a model's hair. $25,000. For the day.

This was the same time I was opening the first Taya salon. In fact, I met Taya at that commercial shoot. We ended up going out to dinner, eating things I wouldn't normally have gotten near, and when it was over, he took my name. For seven years.

Needless to say, I loved Tokyo, Japan.

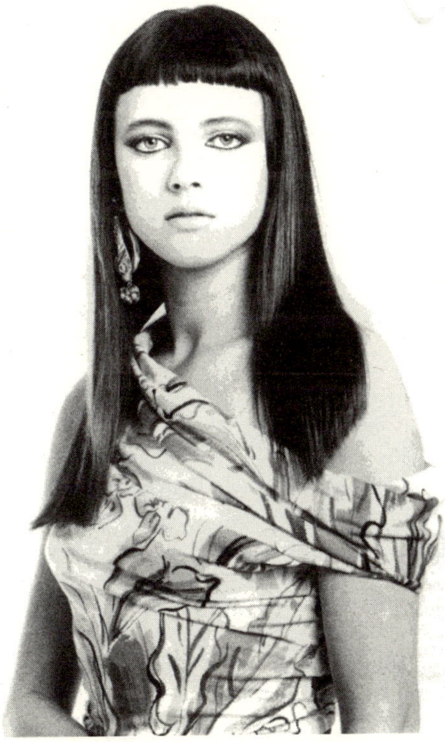

I also ended up experiencing the nightlife in Japan. I had an assistant on that commercial shoot, and he took me out at night. We went to a seven-story warehouse called Gold. It was a nightclub. One of the wildest places I'd ever been. Each floor had a different theme. By three in the morning, there were Japanese girls passed out all over the place. I thought I'd died and gone to Asian heaven.

My relationship with Lux continued. They called me frequently to do their commercials and introduced me to a rising young star named Jennifer Connelly. The first commercial was great. The second one… not so great. The Japanese wanted her to have extremely curly hair. Problem:

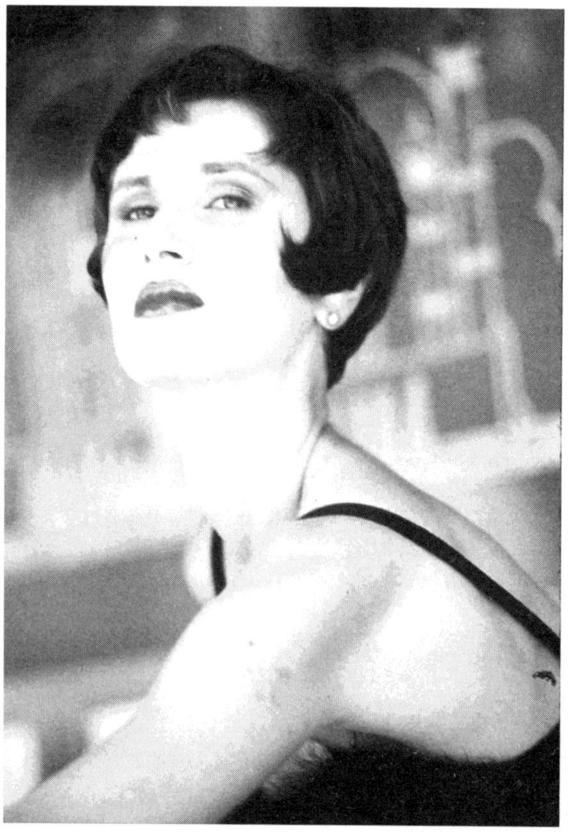

her hair was stick-straight. They kept sending me pictures of what they thought was curly. Kinky, wavy, crimped. I couldn't figure out what they wanted.

One day, I was so frustrated I muttered, "Why don't they just hire a model with curly hair?"

Jennifer heard me. Our relationship changed. She became cold and aloof, not that she was ever that warm and friendly. I took her aside and asked her what was wrong. She told me. I apologized, telling her that it had absolutely nothing to do with her. Basically I kissed her feet. As any great hairdresser would do.

The shoot ended up going beautifully (finally). And she used me again in New York for a magazine ad they were doing.

At the photographers' studio, her hair needed to be blown straight. I started blowing her hair out and it started sticking to her head like glue.

"What's wrong with my hair?" she asked.

I felt like I was about to faint.

I went into the bathroom and splashed some water on my face, praying to God for some guidance. God in his infinite wisdom yelled, "VELCRO ROLLERS."

He really did. Really.

I set her hair in Velcro rollers, and from that moment on I believed in God completely.

Back to Reality and Beverly Hills

I remember sitting in the living room with Lisa one night. My feet were up on the table and I had a beer in one hand, my career in the other. I'm sure I had this glazed look on my face. I know my ears weren't working too well because she practically had to shout my name before I heard her.

"What?" I asked.

"What are you going to do?" she said in a normal tone of voice. The dog was curled up on the floor at her feet. Every once in a while he'd lift his head to look at her, give me a sideways glance, yawn and then lay his head back down with a sigh.

"That's how I feel, buddy," I muttered. I'm sure he was thinking "Great, just what we need is another freakin' drama."

"What?" Now it was Lisa's turn to ask the innocuous question.

"He just seems r-r-r-re-resigned."

She looked at me with concern. She was still sick at this point. The doctors hadn't yet diagnosed her Chronic Fatigue Syndrome. She hadn't had her implants removed. She was huddled on the couch in her favorite sweats and slippers. She looked tired. She looked beautiful. She always looked beautiful. She still does.

"You're stuttering," she said.

"I'm tired."

"You don't usually stutter around me."

"I said I'm tired."

"You've been tired around me, too."

I sighed like the dog and took a swig from my beer. The wind was blowing outside; that wicked, destructive Santa Ana wind that can whip Southern California into a frenzy. Branches snapped off trees and landed on cars, setting off alarms. The house creaked. The kids were off in their rooms, playing some kind of music. My head hurt.

"I have a meeting with Jerry in the morning," I said. She nodded ever so slightly and continued to watch me. I could see the concern in her eyes, and I knew it was about more than the fact I was tired. Or that my little empire I had so painstakingly built was beginning to crumble. The Jerry-in-the-morning was my lawyer, Jerry Chizever. We were going to talk. I felt like I was going to see my father after crashing the car the night before. Talk. It was such an ominous word.

I finished my beer and went to bed. I slept hard and woke up early. It was going to be a very bad day.

Allen and his terrible, horrible, no good, really shitty day

I slouched in the chair in my office in my Beverly Hills salon. My pride and joy. My claim to fame. If you had a salon in Beverly Hills, you were something. I was something. I was a success.

I was about to receive a body blow that would knock me to the mat. I wasn't sure I'd be able to get up. I could see myself, like a short, lightweight prizefighter, dancing around the ring, my eyes blackened, my lip bleeding, holding up my gloves to fend off my opponent. Then I got clocked with a left I didn't see coming.

"You're losing it," Jerry said.

I could see the words hanging in the air like a dialogue balloon from a cartoon. "The Beverly Hills salon… well, you can't afford it. You've got a $1 million lease and no hairdressers. You've got Irvine and Woodland Hills, plus two others. I don't see how you can stay in Beverly Hills. You're hemorrhaging hairdressers; you've got no staff."

He paused. Then went for the jugular: "Allen. Either you lose it or you sell it."

I sat in the chair behind my desk, my back ramrod straight. My head was spinning. It hurt. The business I'd spent so many years building up, the reputation I had painstakingly formulated, my precious Beverly Hills, the crème de la crème of locations, was in flames. All because Paul had decided he didn't want to cut hair anymore. All because I had tried a little product line. All because I had tried to franchise. All because… My decisions were hanging over me like Death with his sickle poised to cut off my head, or some other equally arrogant part of my body. My staff. My hairdressers. Gone. All of it gone, or close to it. Nothing left. I was down to my last few dollars. I actually thought about pulling out my wallet just then, if for no other reason than to show that it wasn't all gone. I had at least a twenty. But if I didn't close Beverly Hills, would I be broke? If I didn't close Beverly Hills, I'd go bankrupt. I knew nothing about bankruptcy. What did it mean? Would I lose everything? This is where my survival instincts kicked in. I was Rambo with a blow dryer, remember?

Lisa and I had talked about this. The other salons were doing well. I'd given up Encino to Paul so that I could keep Beverly Hills. How could it be going under? How could I be going broke because of it?

How?

Everything had been jamming, and now all of a sudden it was going, going, soon to be gone. It was like being blind-sided… I had bought out Paul, my partner, because I knew that with Lisa as my partner, we could do it and do it better together. That, and Paul just plain pissed me off. I had given him the Encino salon as part of the deal. But now Beverly Hills was worthless, it had a million dollar lease, and all I could think was: "I have nothing. My empire's crumbling and Paul's got a new salon in Encino."

"You're going to have to give it all up, Allen."

It hit me then. I was about to become everything that I had vowed I would never be. Like my father before me, who never achieved the success that I'm sure he dreamed of, I felt like a failure. My father's face passed before my eyes. It was a tired, ragged face. Kind, but disappointed. Worn down by the years and lack of drive and desire to truly change his life. I was going to be different than my father.

I was going to rock the world. I had rocked the world. Now the world was rocking back.

Sitting there in my office, I could smell the fragrance of the salon, shampoos and hairspray co-mingling with the chemicals of perms and color. I could hear the silence, the deafening silence of the missing hairdressers and their clients. I still dream of having empty salons and no hairdressers.

You're going to have to give it all up, Allen.

"No, I-I-I-I." I stopped.

Miserable fucking stutter. It always seemed to come back to me when I was faced with a situation over which I felt I had no control. You're. Giving. Up. I was becoming the loser I was afraid of.

"I'm not," I said.

My lawyer looked at me with a quizzical look.

"I'm not giving it up," I said.

And then I smiled.

"You know what? Fuck it. I've still got my name."

And in the salon business, that's everything.

That's the image.

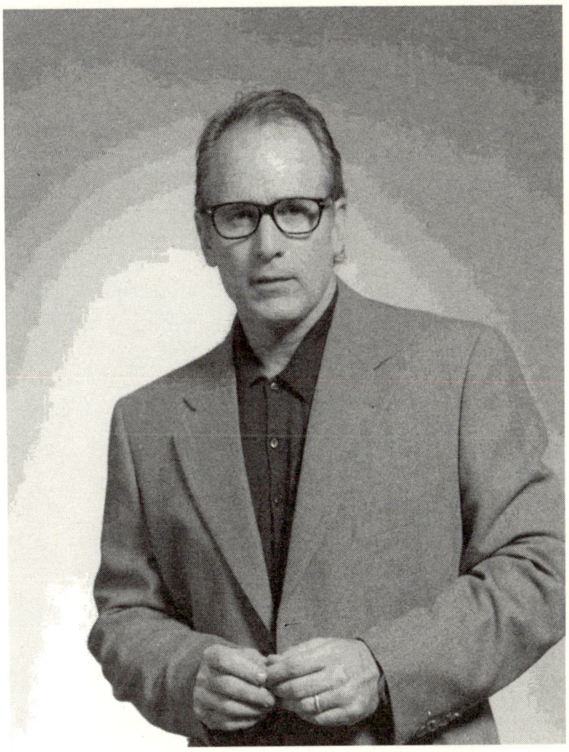

Me as Clark Kent.

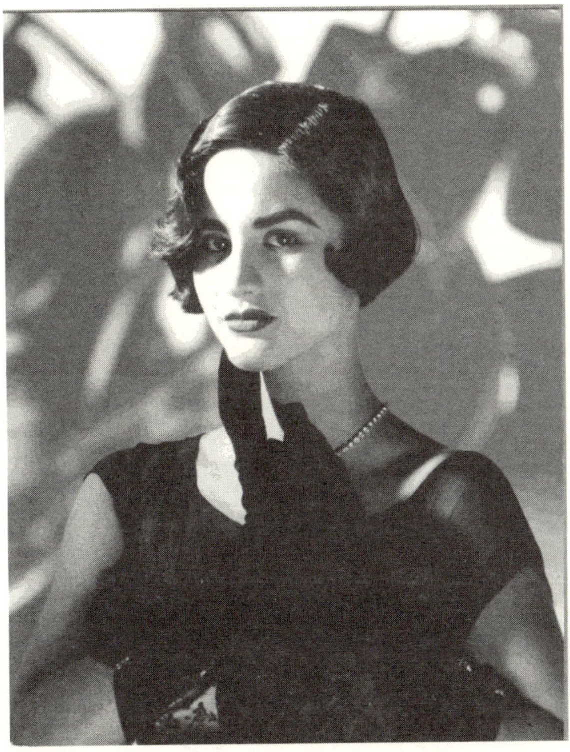

Thinking like Allen.
That's the image.

The Image-Maker

What's that old saying? When you get to the end of your life, you probably won't say you wish you'd spent more time at the office. In my case, the salon. Except… maybe I will. I've always been an image-maker. I was born to be an image-maker.

I look back at my time behind the chair and I realize how much I've seen. How much I've created. Amazing stuff. God, I really am good.

It all started for me in the 1960s. I know that American glamour really started in the 1920s, but it was all about high society then. In the 1960s, high society went mainstream. Rich people weren't the only ones who had style and image.

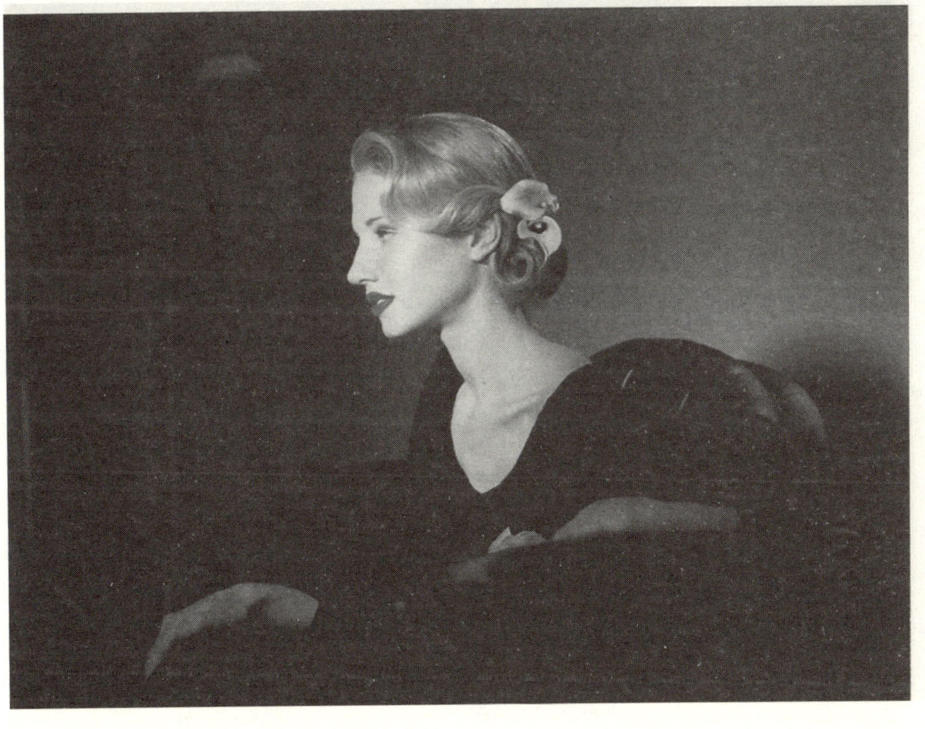

In the 1950s, women didn't work very much. It was still the era of the hairdo. Women wanted to look good for their husbands when they came home after a hard day at the office. Women got their hair done at the beauty parlor, going at least once a week for the glamour. Film and television were a huge influence, as they still are, making glamour very accessible. Non-glamorous people wanted to be glamorous people; they wanted to emulate them. It's a law of nature. The everyday housewife wanted to look like Ginger Rogers, Lauren Bacall. Women set and teased their hair, went for the up-do. This was during the Elvis flip, the bubble, the big tease.

In 1950s French movies, the hair was cut, not teased. I think Europe has always been a little bit ahead of us. Think *Funny Face* and Audrey Hepburn, where she sat in a beauty parlor and had all her hair cut off. Suddenly women wanted to do that, they wanted to be that daring. They wanted to be Audrey Hepburn. Women then were great followers.

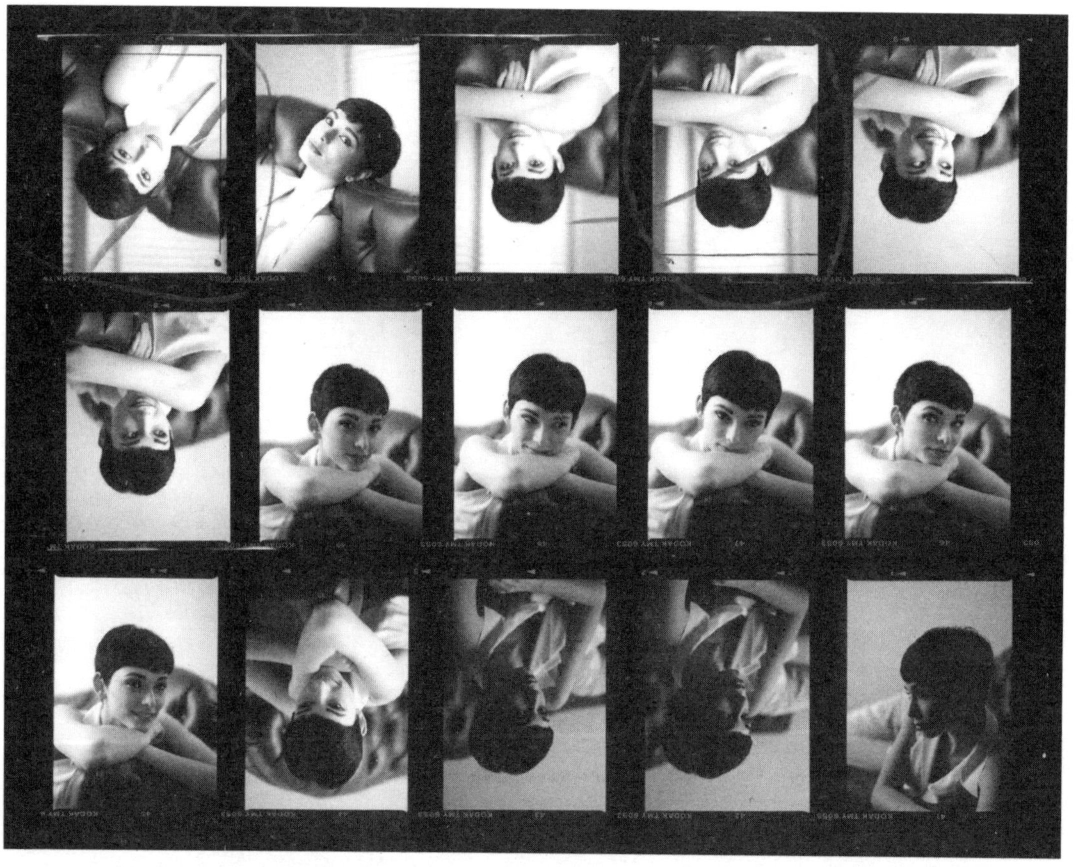

It was Europe that first started using the blow dryer. The French were really starting to cut hair. We were still wrapped up in the hair-wrapped-in-toilet-paper phase, with paper clips on the side curls. The hair was always sprayed with pure lacquer. Beehives were up so long that spiders were living in them. This was helmet hair. I could have worn that kind of hair on my motorcycle and it would have protected me. Men's styles were ducktails and jellyrolls. Nerds had little parts and waves in the front with really short sides.

And then, of course, came the 1960s and the Beatles. The longhaired lads from Liverpool. There was such negativity about men having long hair. It was epitomized by *Easy Rider*, where the characters played by Peter Fonda and Dennis Hopper were killed for going into the South with long hair. Could men's hair get longer? You bet.

Jay Sebring started doing a lot with men's hair. He virtually created men's styling. It was the era of the pompadour, where everything was cut short and even. I'm talking men here. They'd cut, put a hair net on and spray it with something Jay called Presto. Think Bob Eubanks.

Jay Sebring unfortunately became much more famous for his death. He was killed, with his friend Sharon Tate, in the famous Helter Skelter murders in a house at the top of Benedict Canyon in Los Angeles, just south of Mulholland Highway.

In these adventurous 1960s there was choice, always something new. One of the top hairdressers was Gene Shacove. He was the innovator of the Joey Heatherton and other famous starlets. Women started changing their looks and then changing them again. Jane Fonda's shag was the beginning. Then bang—everyone wanted to cut their hair like Jane Fonda. Finally, the rollers were being put away.

It ushered in unconstructed, loose looks. This was when Vidal Sassoon first arrived on the scene and started emphasizing the cut. No more set, no more tease. Hairdressers started using blow dryers. They were becoming more stylists and had to relearn how to cut hair all over again. Women started doing their hair at home. They started washing it and conditioning it. The salons weren't as necessary.

But all that meant was that hairdressers had to invent new ways to do things. New ways of cutting, of styling. We had to invent new looks. Like Sassoon did with the Twiggy, and like I did with the Farrah. We created shags, geometrics, punk, and styles like the bob that changed by the day.

The fun thing was to create. I mean, I did one of the most famous haircuts in the world. But my doing it didn't make it famous. The hair being exposed on *Charlie's Angels* every week is what made it famous. The bikinis didn't hurt.

Enter the 1970s. Hair had started to get bigger, with both Farrah and Cher. Hair was all about sex. While the 1960s were about experimentation, war and drugs, the '70s were about wild sex and wild abandon. Women finally realized that they could have sex without being in love, and it was OK. They wore push-up bras, poor-boy tops, bell-bottoms, platform shoes.

This experimentation reached women who had never been glamorous before, and it gave them a chance to look like a movie star. It wasn't dramatic. It was a haircut. Suddenly, girls everywhere wanted to be Farrah. It gave them identity, something different than what they had. They identified with the beauty. Let's face it. Some people aren't beautiful, but every woman has the ability to bring out her own beauty. And they can have beautiful, sexy hair. When they have beautiful hair, they start feeling good about themselves.

You want to feel good? Change your hair. It's the only thing on your body that you can cut off. It's not permanent. You can change it and change it, and then change it again.

The wedge was one of the most interesting haircuts ever designed. When Dorothy Hamill won the gold at the Olympics, everybody wanted the wedge. The problem was, it was a difficult look to put on most women. It looked good on Dorothy because she was twirling around all the time. When she spun around, the world went spinning-wedge crazy. Even though most people didn't look good with it, hairdressers loved to cut it. It was fun. And you can't cut a sloppy wedge. Problem: most women don't spin their way through life, so the Dorothy Hamill just sort of hung.

The 1980s was one of the sexiest times for hair. Big curly hair, like what Cher wore in her music video—you know, the one where she straddled the cannon on the aircraft carrier in San Diego—opened up a whole new world of fashion.

Perms with 200 rods. Big shoulders, bigger hair. Power hair. Think Donna Mills on *Knots Landing*, Joan Collins and Linda Evans on *Dynasty*.

Every year there was a new look, and it was always fun.

Hair somehow always comes to define an era

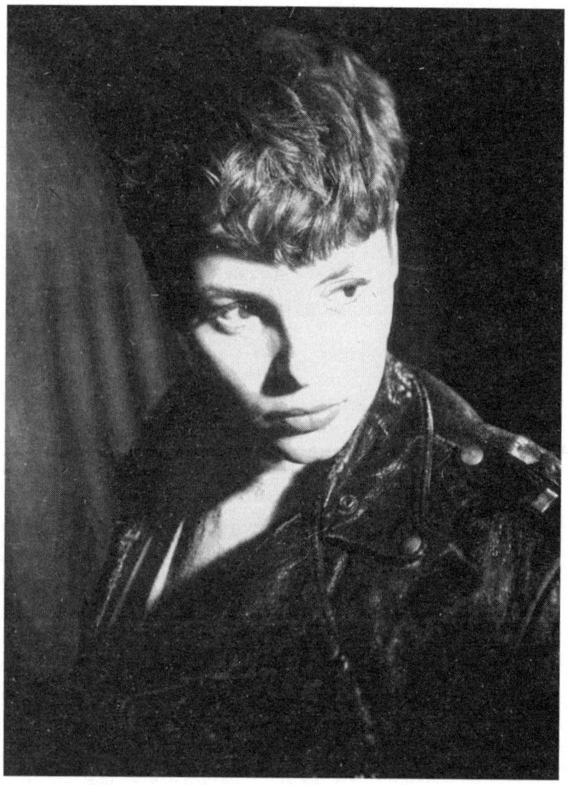

Think about the 1950s.

Grease. The tough guy with the jelly-roll. Every stereotype had a look: the jock with the flat top, crew cut and letterman jacket; the greaser with the leather motorcycle jacket and boots (think Marlon Brando, and John Travolta in *Grease*—again with the Travolta). Levi's were worn by everybody. The Latinos wore split khakis, serge shirts, wing-tip shoes. Those were interesting. They had such high shine you could comb your hair by looking in them. Hair was very one-length, slicked back.

I always felt that the Latinos had a great sense of style. I loved how they put their outfits together, starting with the Zoot suits in the 1940s. They also had great cars, with the low-riders. Today, it's done with hydraulics. In the old days they torched the springs. Gotta ride low.

But people have always been looking for change. From the 1950s to the 1980s, there was always a new look, a new must-have. That's because there were new things. Constantly. New cars, bigger and flatter televisions, smaller music players. The American dream. Every six months hair responded to another trend. It still does.

In the '50s, '60s and '70s, women were big hair followers. If a movie star changed her hair, the women followed. Even Lucille Ball trended with her red hair.

Haircuts had names and personalities then, like the dances of the '60s. The Jane Fonda shag, Mia Farrow and Twiggy with the wedge. The twist, the pony, the skate, the watoosi.

We don't name the cuts anymore. They're the celebrities. The Farrah. The Jennifer Aniston. The Beckham. There are so many celebrities today. TV stars are as big as movie stars. Sometimes bigger.

When Donna Mills cut her long hair, when she was doing *Knots Landing*, everyone wanted the same look. It was relatable, especially because she was on television. By being on television, she became someone that everyone thought they knew. She became a friend, or in the case of Abby, her character, a nemesis. Still, it explains why Jennifer Aniston was such a phenomenon on *Friends*. She became a friend to millions.

With the Donna Mills cut another new trend emerged: scrunching. It was a phenomenon. No setting, no roller brushes, no geometrics. Cut it, flip it and squeeze it. Women loved it. Hairdressers loved doing it. It was easy.

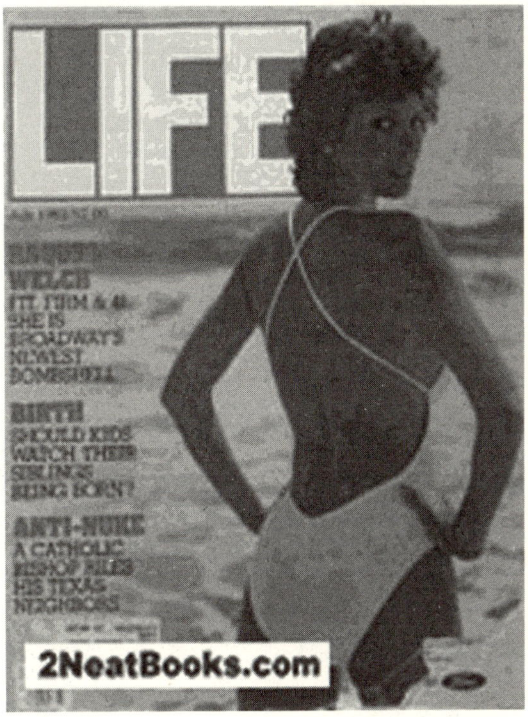

Most actresses change their hair for a part. In the old days, actresses would keep their style for years. It became their signature. They were afraid to change because they wouldn't be the same anymore. A good example is Raquel Welch. When she first came to me, she had long, sexy hair. But she wasn't 21 anymore. When she hit 40, she went out for a part and couldn't get it because of her age. She got pissed off. She came to me. We cut her hair off short and she was a new woman. She went to New York and did the Broadway play *Woman of the Year*. I'm not saying it was only because of her hair, but the hair helped. Today's stars change their hair like they change their underwear. If they're wearing underwear.

OK. They also change their hair for a character.

Even music stars get in the act. Who would have thought that the big-hair rockers of the 1980s would cut off all their hair? Look at Motley Crue or Bon Jovi. David Lee Roth. Even Elton John changes his toupees. They're almost respectable. It keeps them new and young.

Madonna is the ultimate image-maker. She changes and redesigns herself to be constantly reborn. So does Prince. Even Michael Jackson was a big image-maker at one point. From clothes to hair to makeup. All three of them. Big influences.

1960s

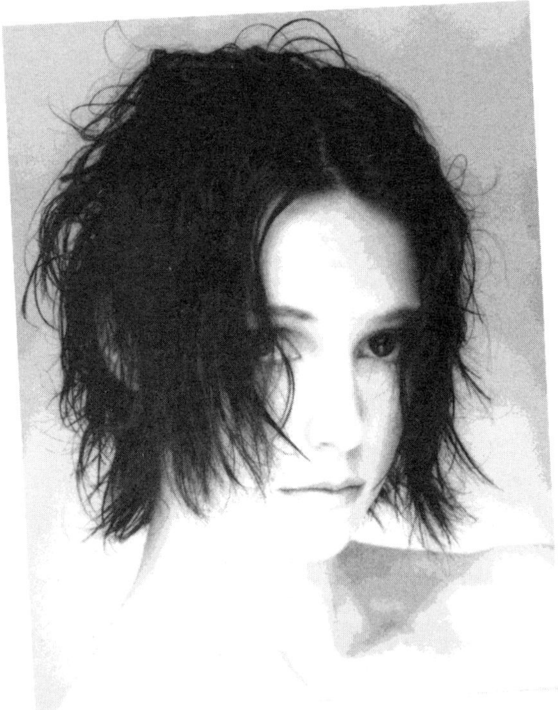

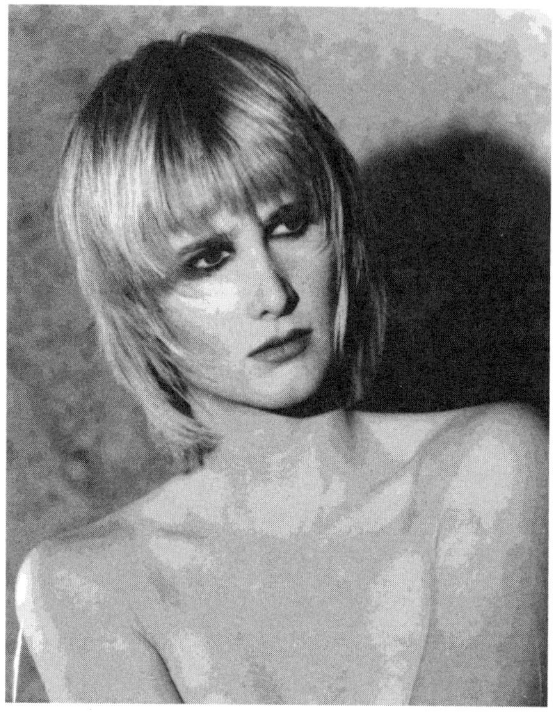

Shags

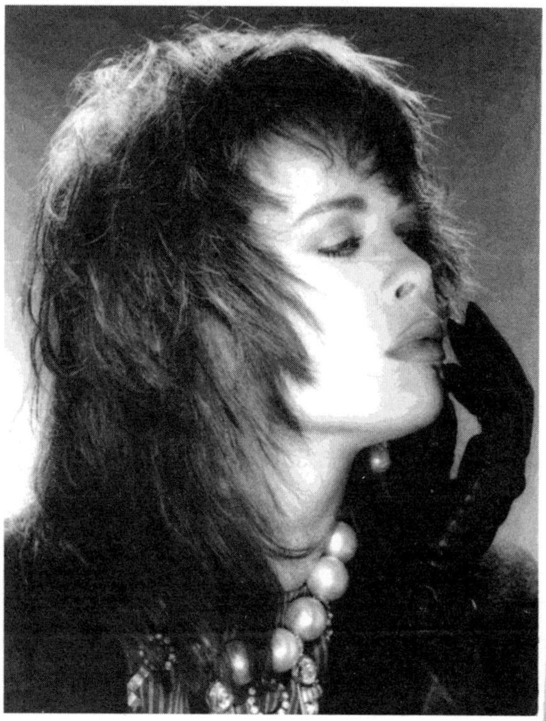

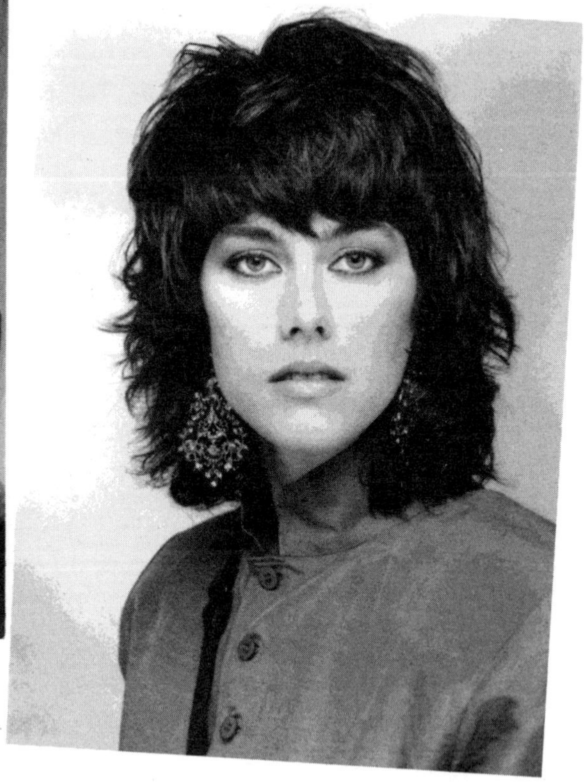

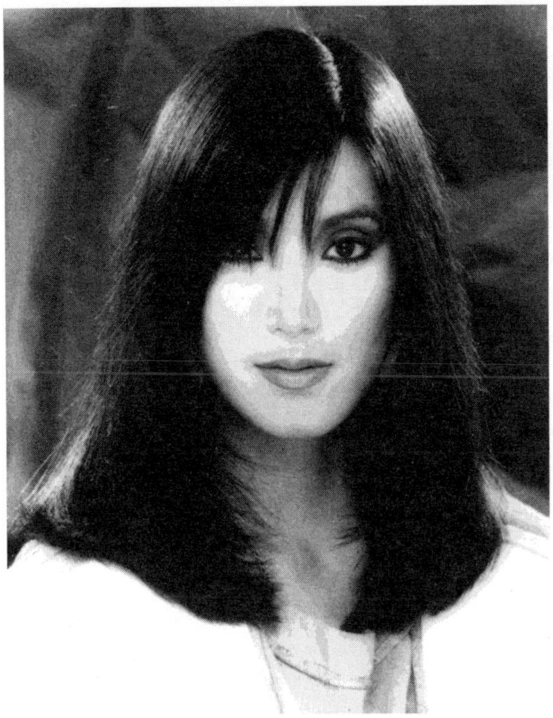

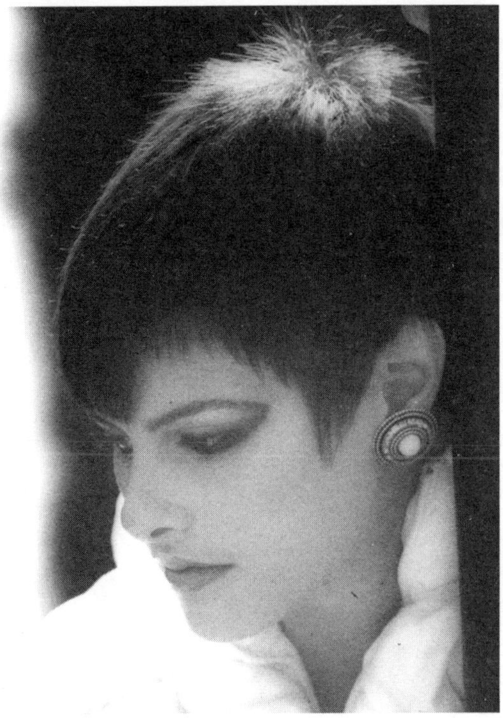

1970s

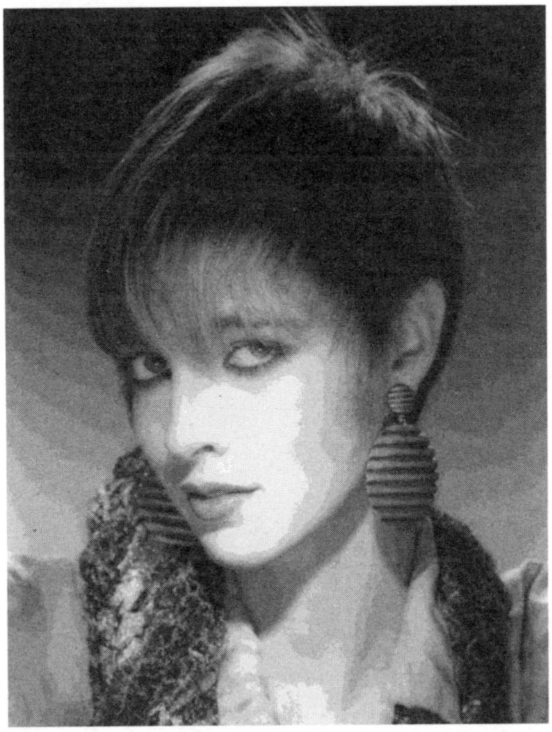

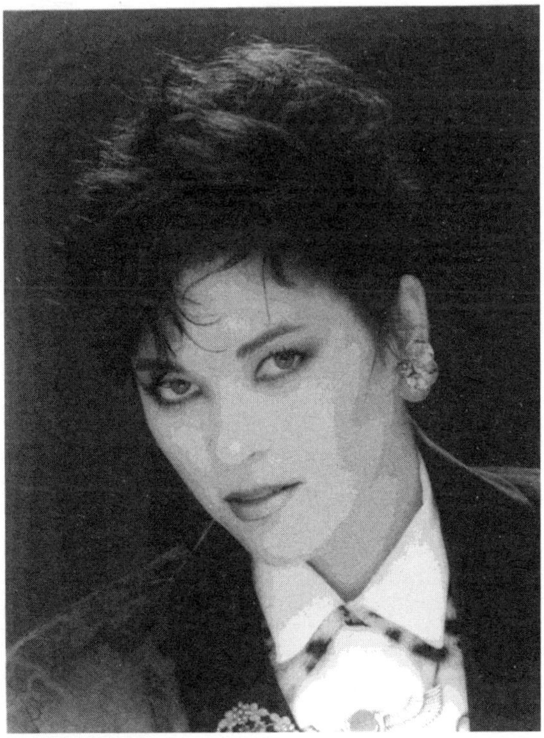

1980s

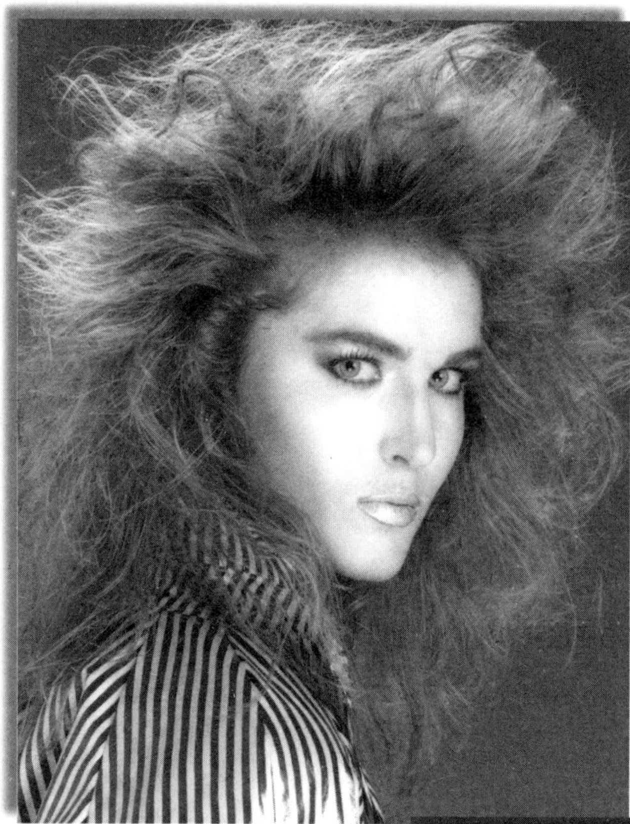

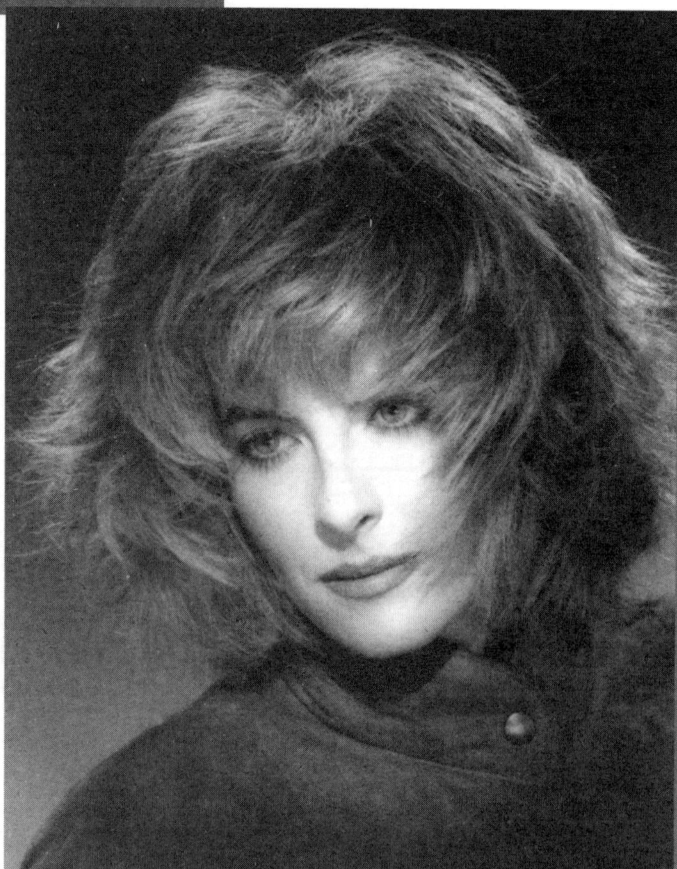

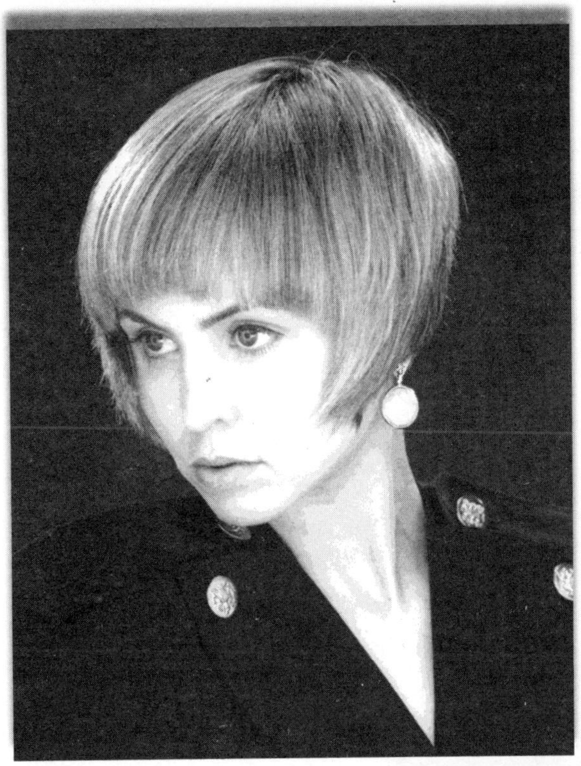

Power hair

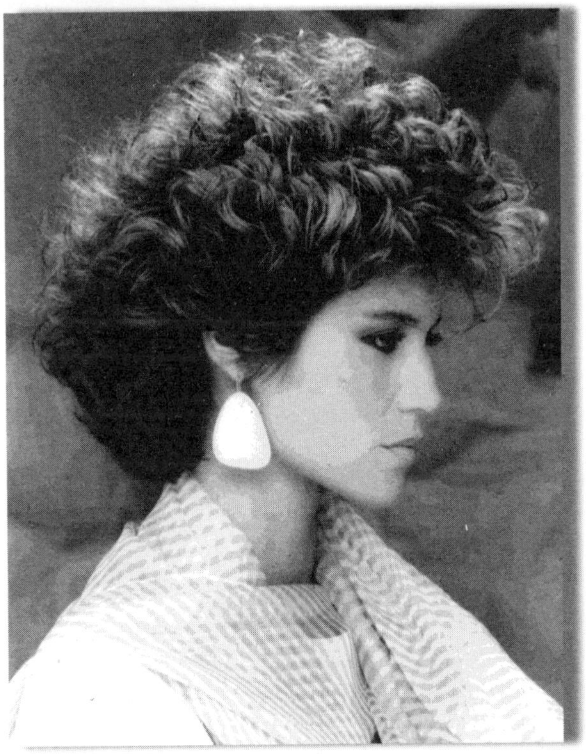

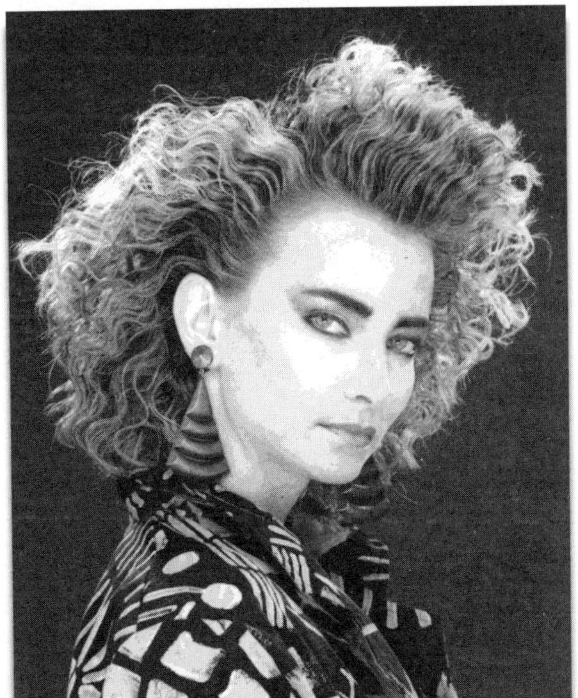

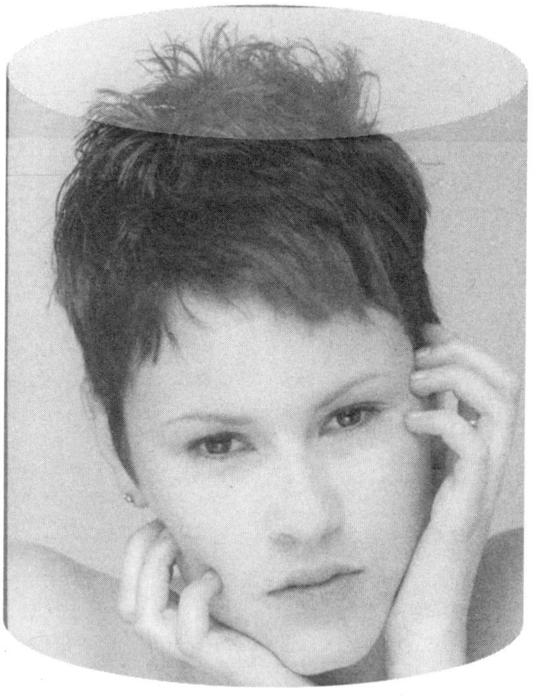

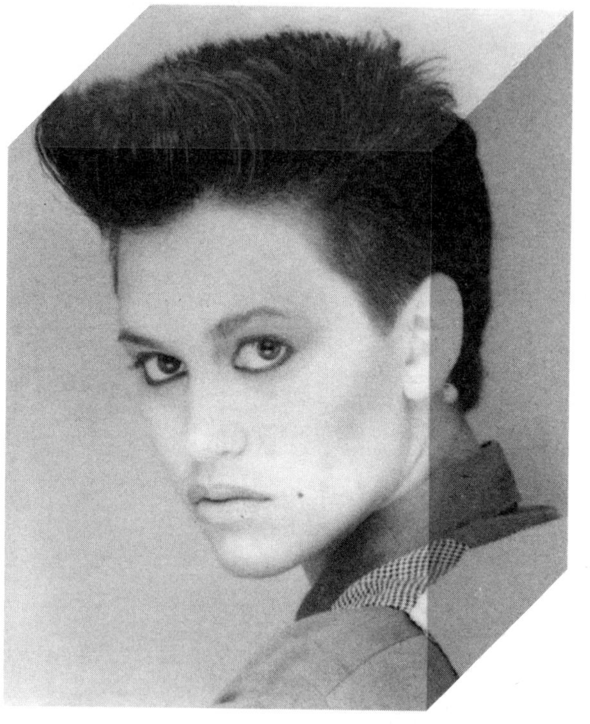

1990s

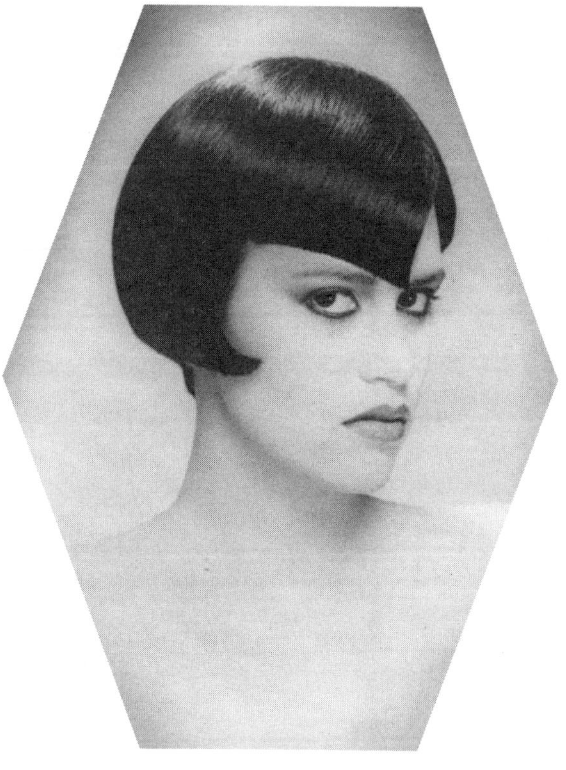

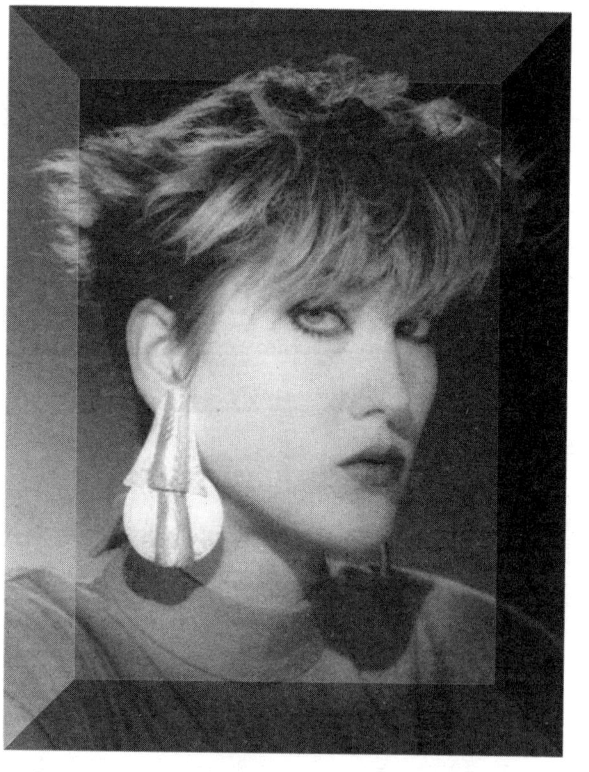

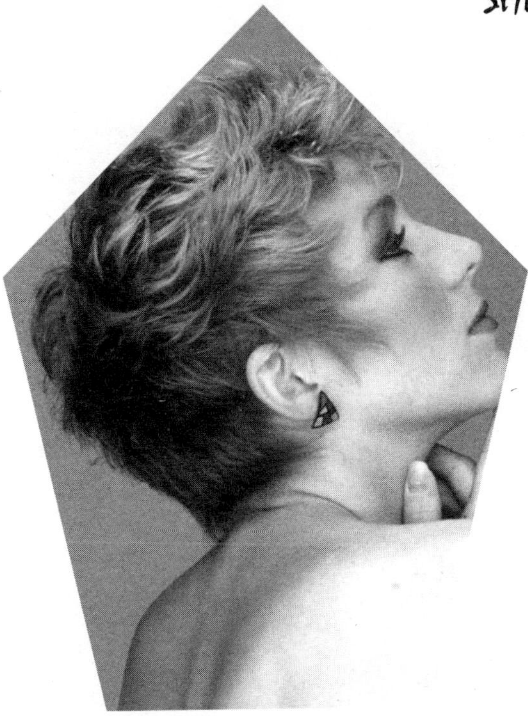

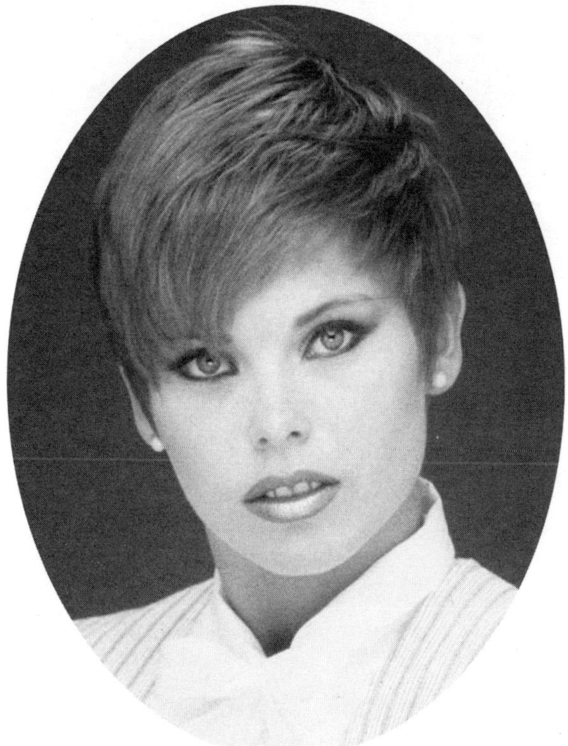

All about the individual

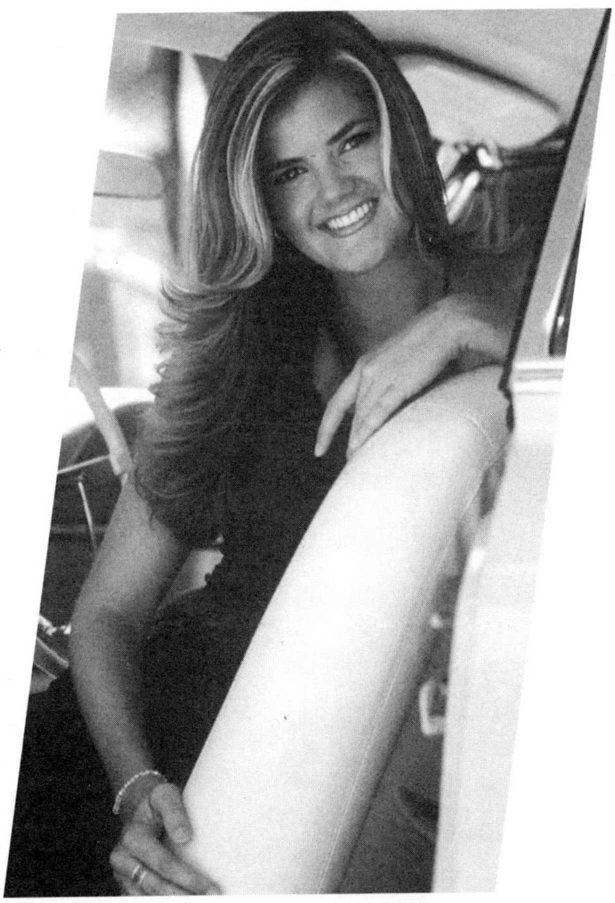

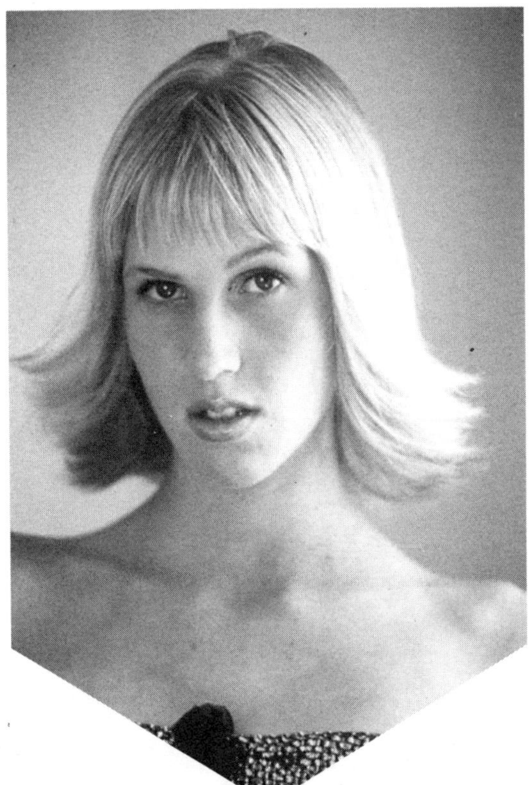

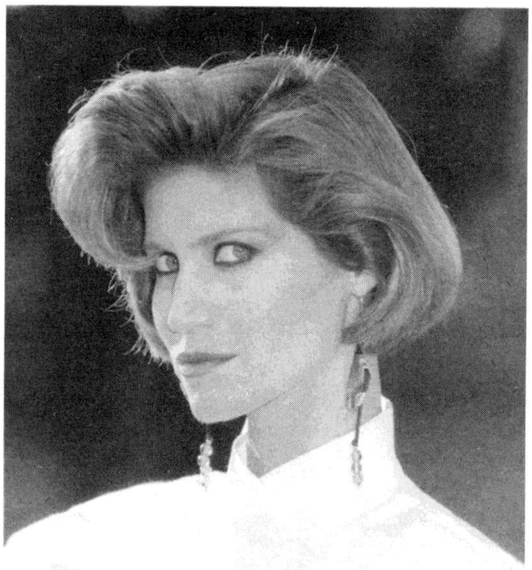

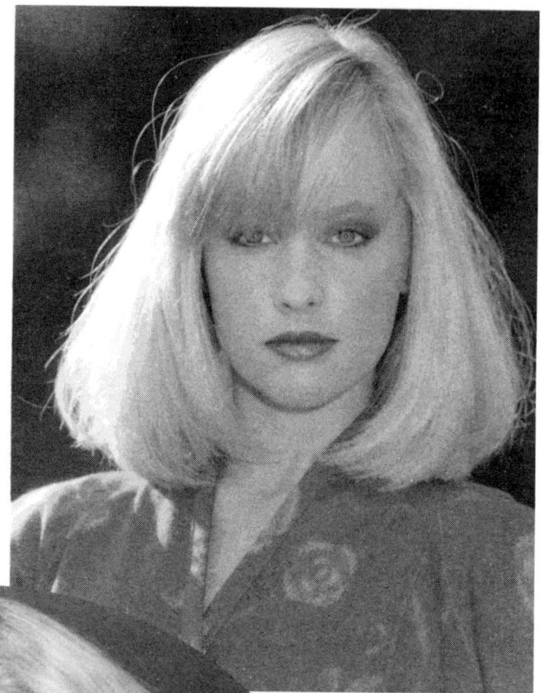

Bobs through

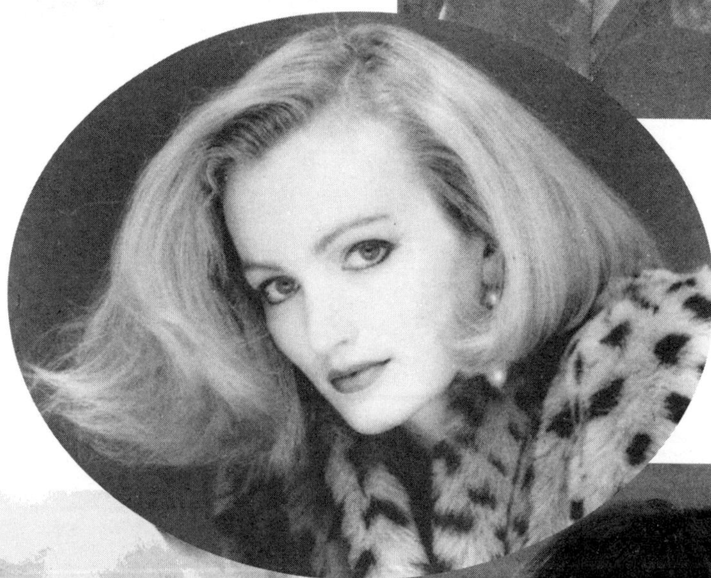

the years

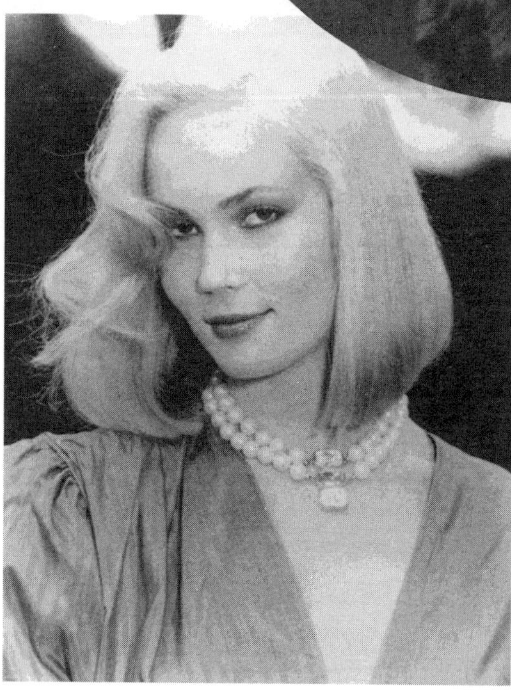

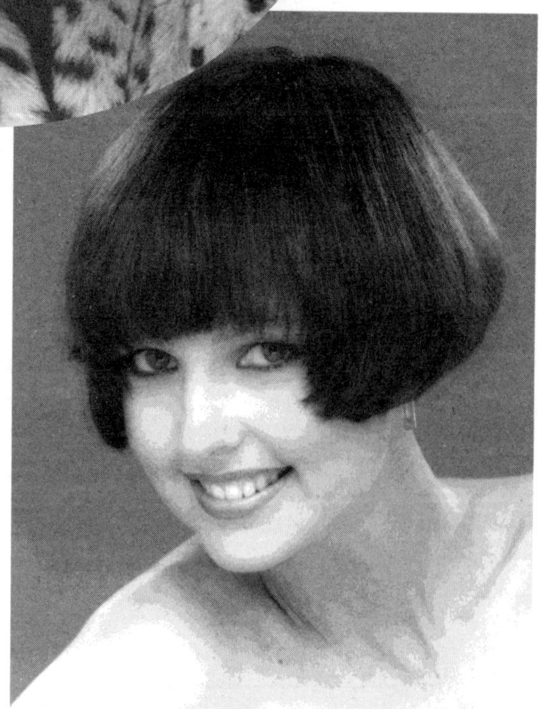

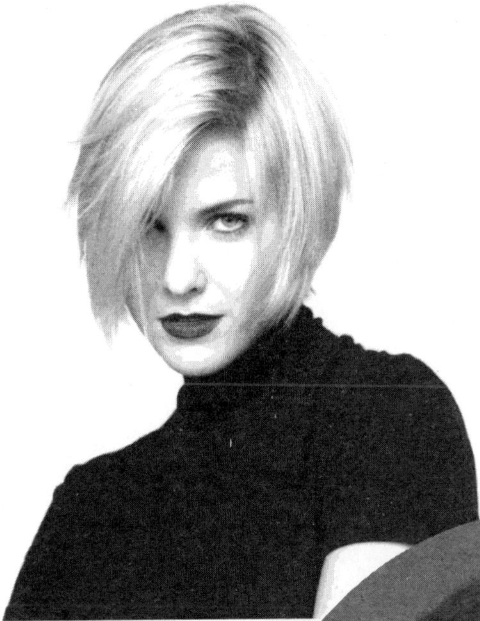

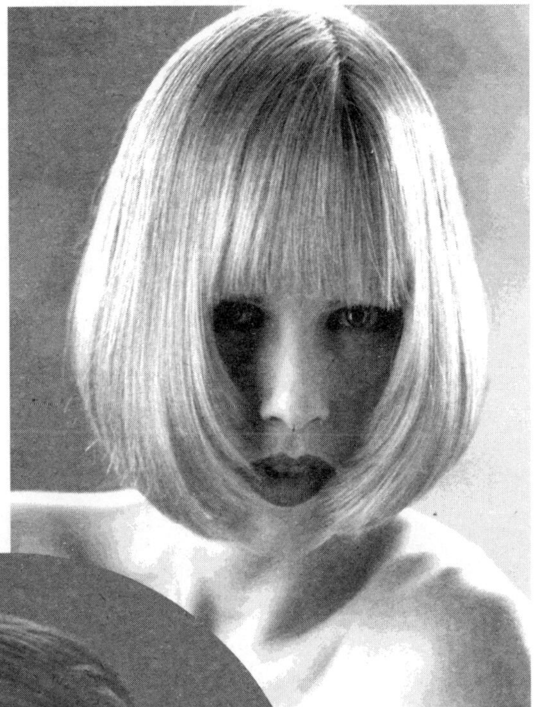

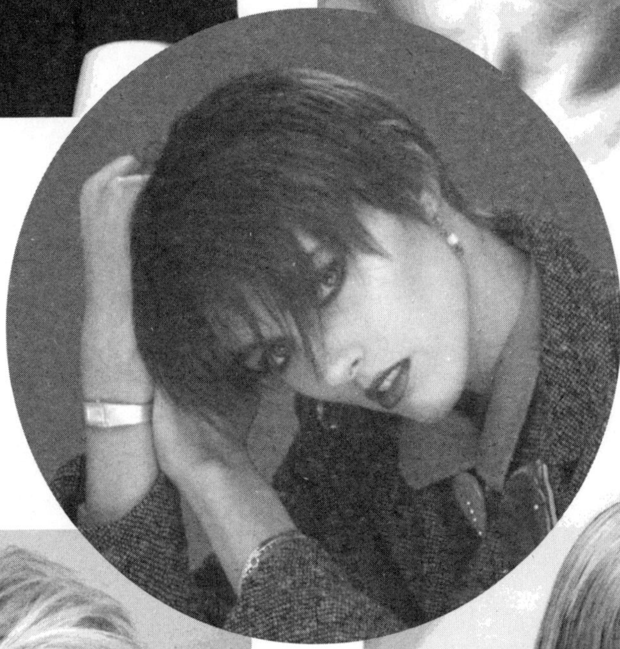

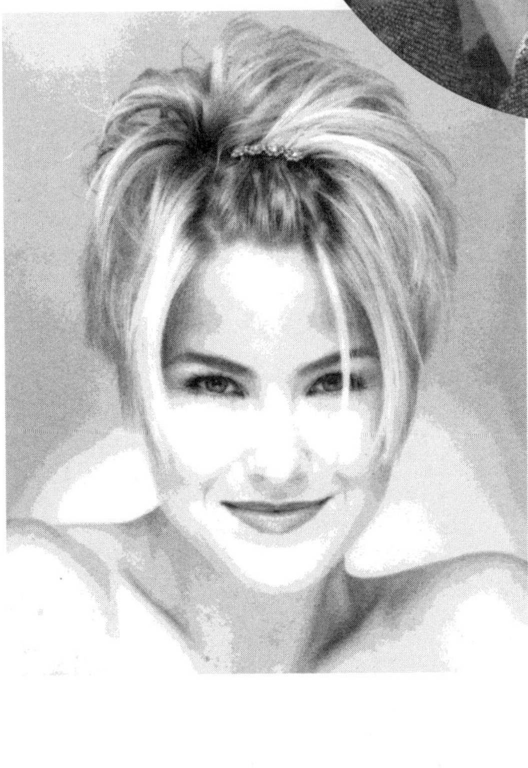

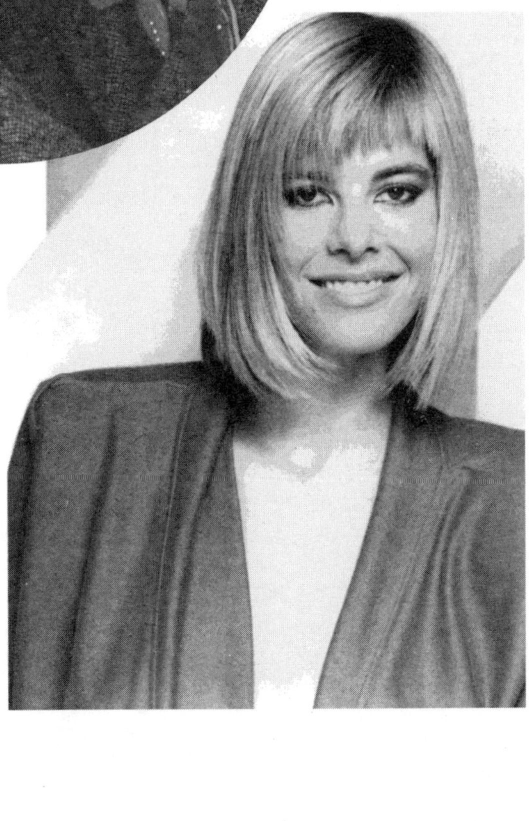

A new century of style

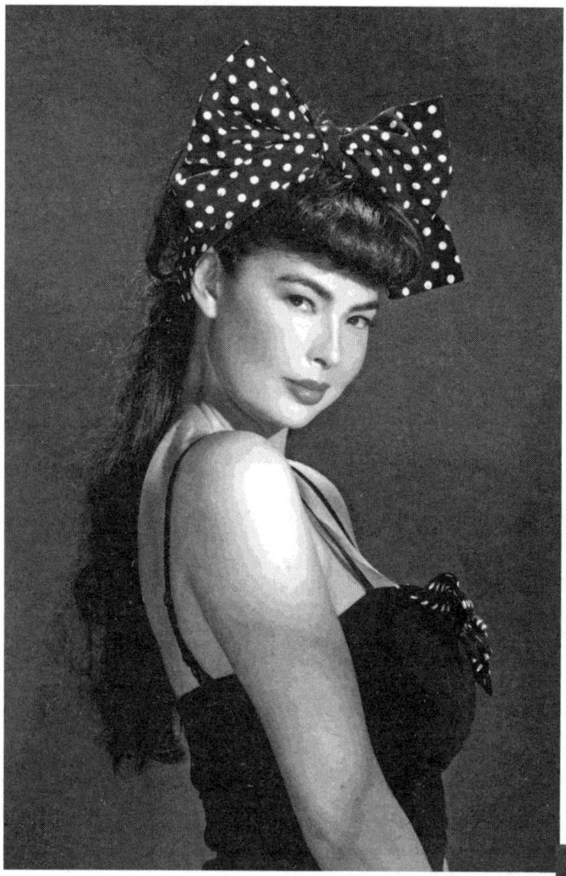

Tara Patrick

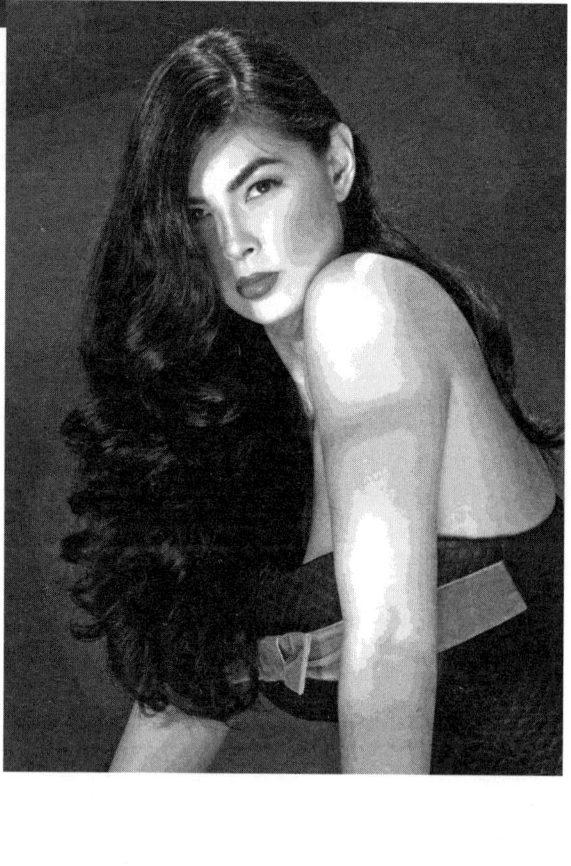

I was always learning new techniques, expanding, reaching. When Sassoon came in the 1960s, things really changed. He was an architect, with a structured way of cutting hair. He actually blueprinted how to cut hair. He'd already been doing it for years in London. He just brought it here. It was only new to us. Hairdressers went crazy over it.

I developed my own technique using tapering scissors, which was handed down from Gene Shacove to Jon Peters to me. We all could make women look sexy and fabulous. Visual freestyle cutting. That's difficult to teach. It's freer, looser. Different than Sassoon. As he was training his geometric, straight sheer perfection cutting, I was teaching how to get in touch with emotions, how to feel the haircut, and to be as creative as possible. I tried doing Sassoon's technique, but it made me feel emotionally blocked and stifled my creatively. That was just me. They'd cut the wedge using a million sections. I could achieve the same look using fewer sections. But using my tapering method, it would come out basically the same, only different. Softer. More fluid.

Because of my technique, I was able to design a cut to suit a personality. I had an ability to make women look really incredible, with something comparable to a Sassoon bob, where sections were blended into each other for perfect imperfection.

I think the reason I mention Sassoon a lot is because I'm truly a fan. Hairdressing is like being an artist. Artists look up to Picasso and Van Gogh. Hairdressers look up to innovators like Sassoon.

Women and their styles and their age

It's important that women don't hang on to a look that they think makes them look younger. As they age, hair should change. They shouldn't hang on to an old look any more than they should wear old-looking clothing styles.

How do I get a woman to recognize that she's hanging onto something old? I just tell her.

Think of it this way: you could go into a dress shop and say, "I'd like something from ten years ago." The clerk will look at you like you're nuts. And you are. Why go into a salon and ask the same thing?

Know your hair. Treat it like an accessory. Have fun. Cut it (which doesn't mean you have to have short hair).

Cut it. The worst that can happen is it will grow back.

In my experience, women will listen to a five-year-old.

"Mommy, don't cut your hair."

Women will listen to their 80-year-old mother.

"Dear, your hair is just fine."

It's keeping you in the same place.

A perfect example is Marcia Clark, the assistant district attorney who prosecuted O.J. Simpson for the murder of his ex-wife and her friend. She started out with a poodle-mullet. Short top with a perm with long, hanging hair in the back. I had a client, Suzanne Childs (very fashionable, very beautiful), who was doing publicity for the DA's office, and she brought Marcia in to see me.

"You have to help," she said. "Can you do something with her hair?"

Marcia sat down in my chair and we talked. I wanted to get a feel for her personality, for what she'd be comfortable with.

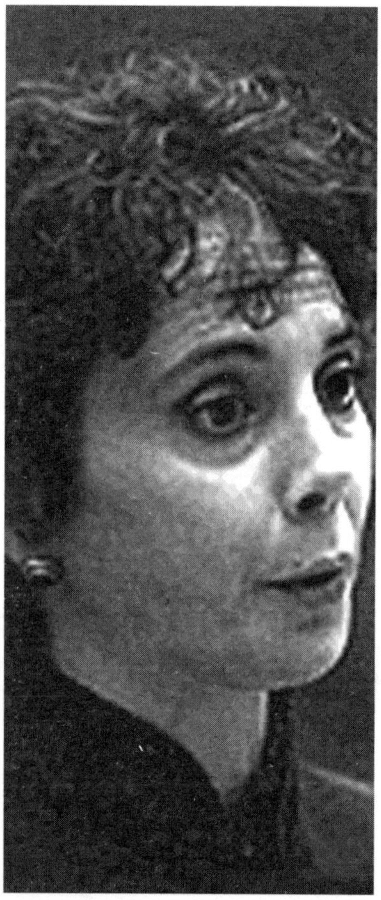

Marcia Clark, before Allen.

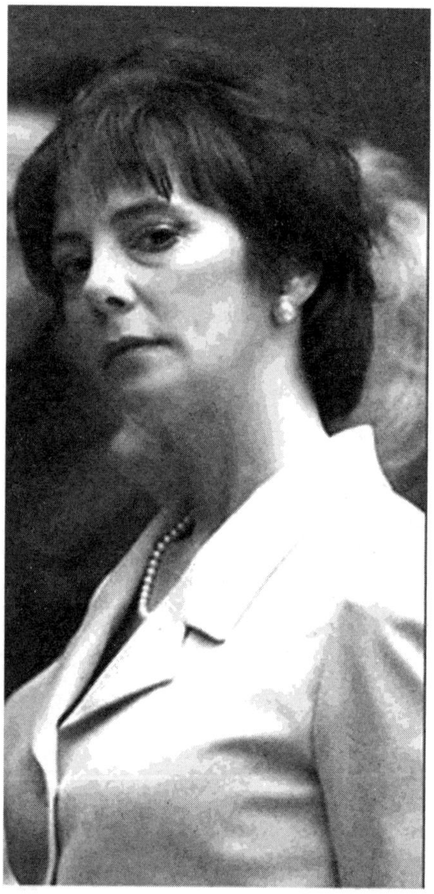

Marcia Clark, after Allen.

Then we CUT IT. Short. Blew it out straight. She went in to court the next day and it was the only thing that got any attention. At least for the day. The reaction was so strong because it looked so much better. It was a simple haircut. It was a big change. The reaction was inappropriate. But it was typical for L.A.

Speaking of L.A., let's talk reality TV

I really believe that TV has change beauty. Especially reality TV, which has made stars out of people who wouldn't (and sometimes shouldn't) have ever been on TV before. Like Jonathon in *Blow Out*. It gave him an opportunity to do something big.

Blow Out was supposed to be about building a hair salon, but it became about the star, his meltdowns and his temper. It betrayed the beauty industry and showcased hairdressers as being dysfunctional. In my humble opinion.

Of course, I had my own dalliance in reality TV with a show called *Split Ends. Split Ends* appeared on the Style network. The idea was to take hairdressers from two different walks of life and switch them. They took famous hairdressers, like me, and shipped us off to little towns in the middle of nowhere. When I was on the show, they sent me to a grandma-neighborhood on Staten Island, New York. You think I'm kidding? On the window was a big sticker that said: Senior Discount $4.

Part of me immediately reverted to my time at Yamanos. I had flashbacks of little old ladies with blue hair, yelling about me because I was just a kid who didn't know anything. Of course, I was nearly 60. In some circles that would have made me a little old man. I didn't want to backtrack. I didn't want to be doing that kind of hair again. So I didn't.

My goal was to get the hairdressers in this salon, who had all worked at one time or another in Manhattan, to raise their game. Change their work. They could still do little old ladies but also do other things. I wanted them to explore the craft.

I truly enjoyed my time there. Switching places, doing something totally foreign, surviving another life for a week. It was a great experience and one of the most fun things I've done in my career. I don't know that the woman who took my place in Los Angeles would say the same thing. She didn't want to change her mindset or learn anything new. She cried every day.

Cable TV has opened doors for hairdressers, makeup artists and tattoo people. And cable TV has created some really big names, like Carson Kressley from *Queer Eye for the Straight Guy*. But the mistake cable reality shows make is hiring people because they do famous people and expecting them to be good because of that fact. It doesn't always work. A perfect example is Sally Hershberger, who's a brilliant hairdresser, but horrible as a judge on *Shear Genius.*

What makes a good haircut?

Start with a consultation. Talk to your hairdresser. Tell him or her what you like and what you don't. Don't get too caught up in star hairdressers. There are great hairdressers all over the country. Find one who fits your needs, whom you can communicate with. You'll have a great relationship. Your cut should be a collaborative process. You have to wear it. Don't be afraid. Believe in the stylist and don't get caught up in the same thing. It might take time to get used to it, but if the hairdresser is truly talented, it will work.

I still cut hair because it's my art. I love it. I like creative haircuts and having a positive response from the person whose hair I just cut. If it's not a positive response, it's not very rewarding. That's what drives me.

Gene Shacove said once: "You can be really good all the time, but it's hard to be phenomenally creative all the time."

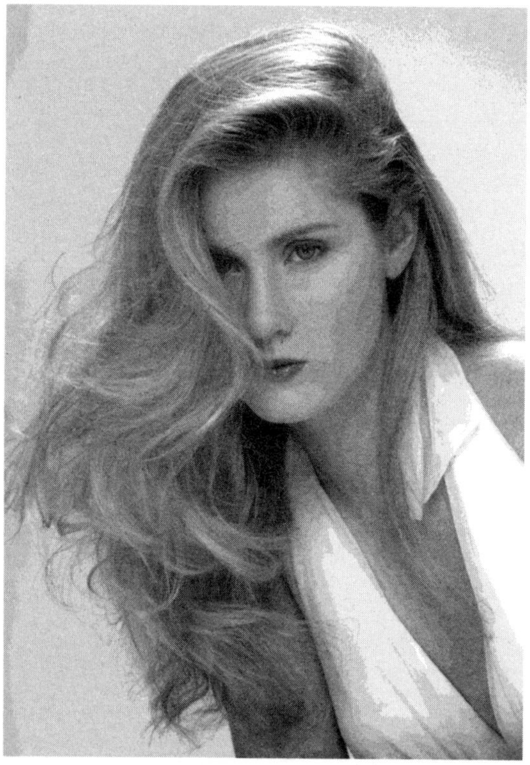

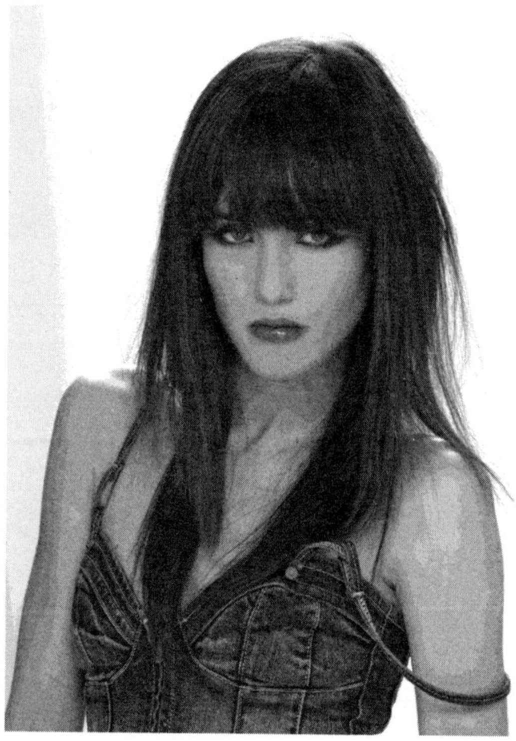

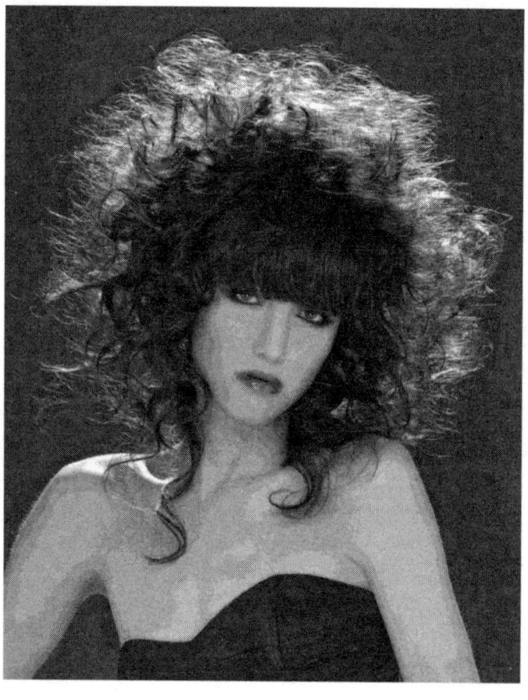

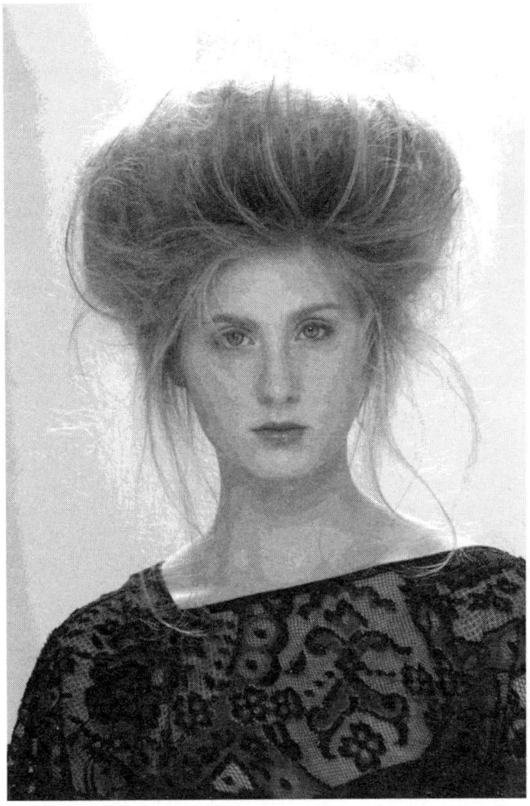

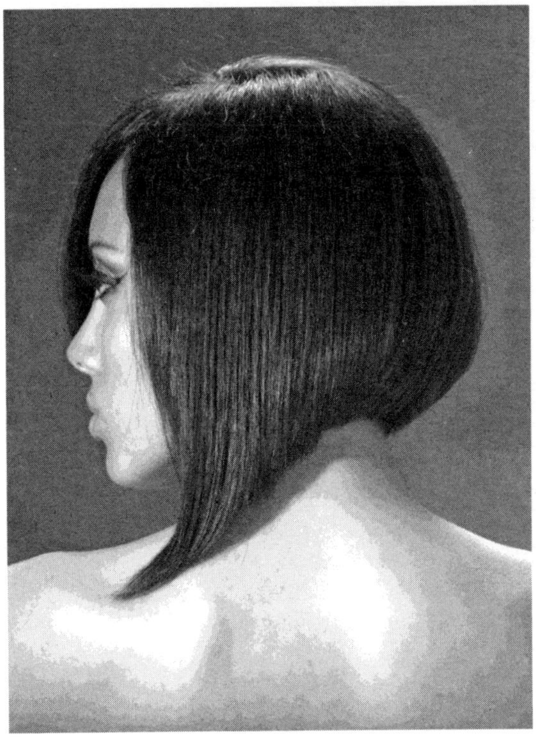

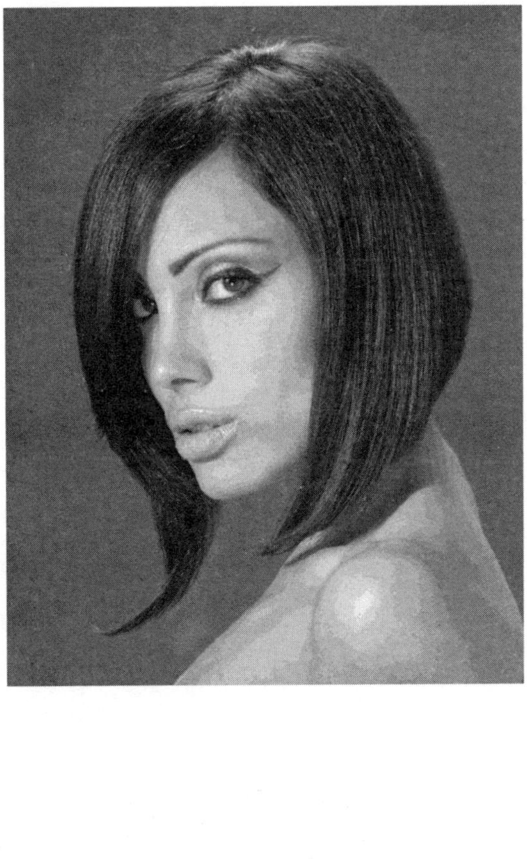

An amazing haircut is done by someone who's connected to his or her art. Get in the zone. That's how I teach my hairdressers. It's about energy.

My energy comes from the haircut turning me on. It's like somebody plugged me in. The excitement is almost sexual. In any kind of art, it's that way. When a client comes back and says, do it again, it's almost impossible. It has to be spontaneous. Like the best sex.

The future won't be any different than it is today. It will just look different. We'll go into the salon to feed the creative monster. We'll be artists.

We'll be image-makers.

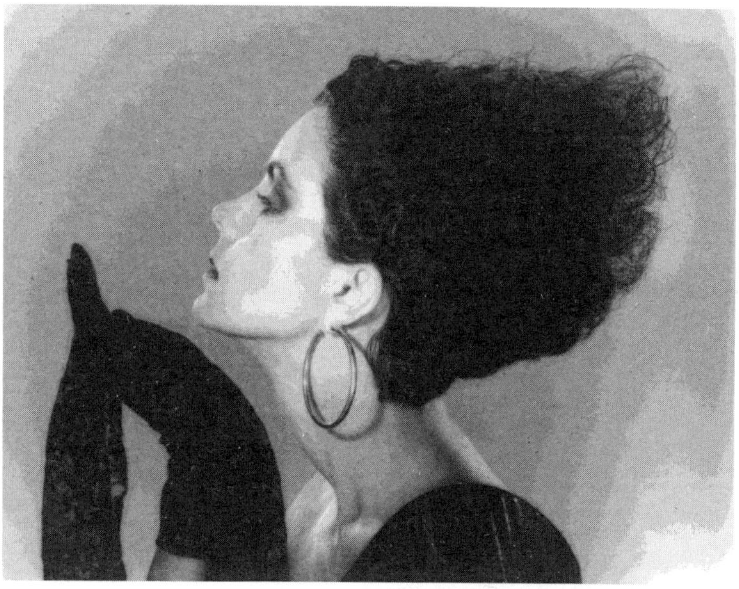

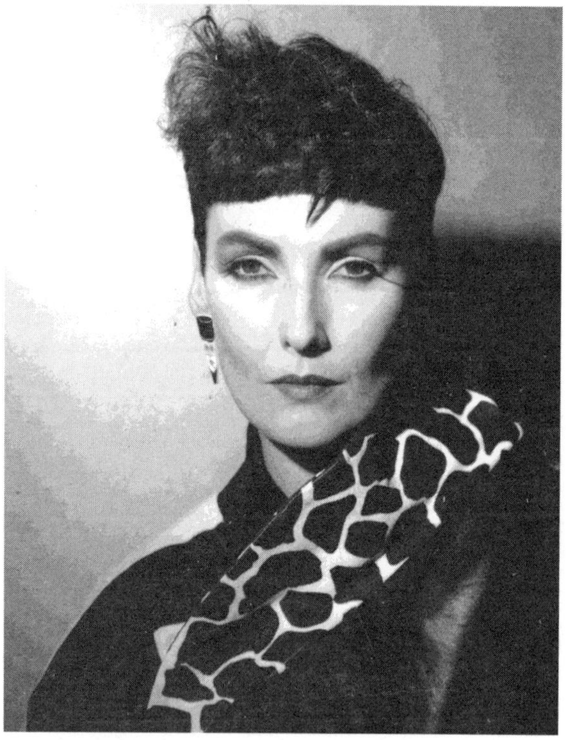

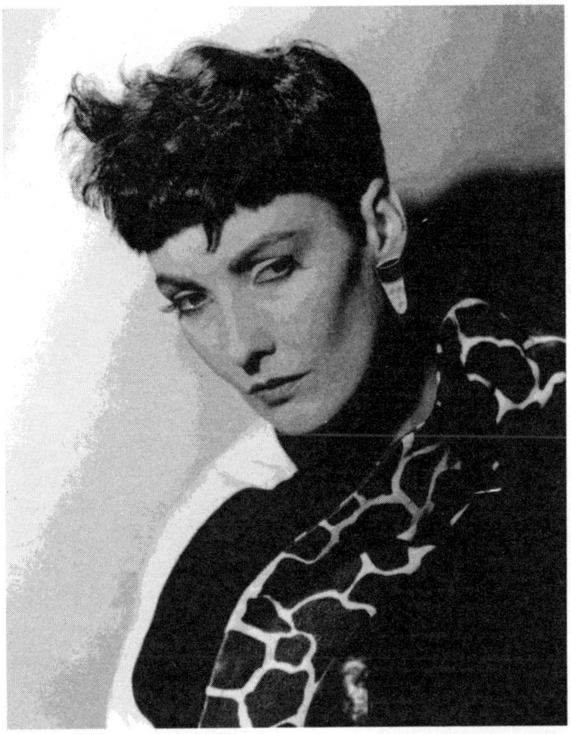

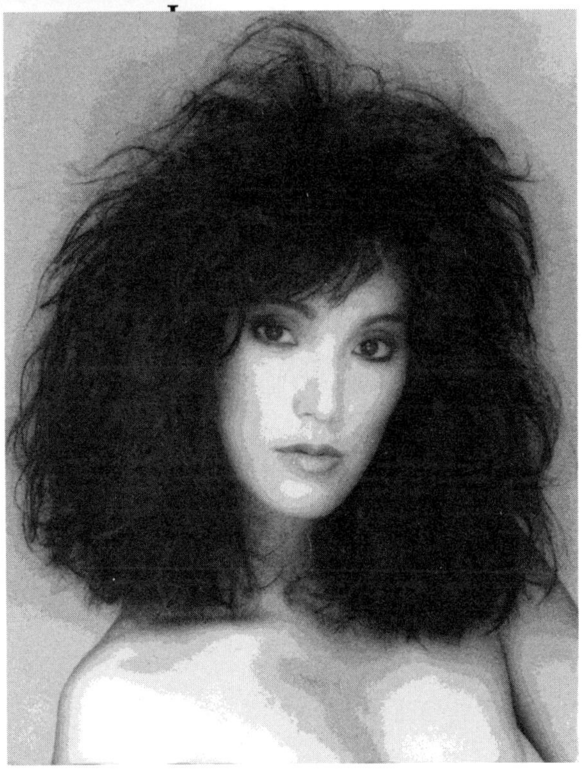

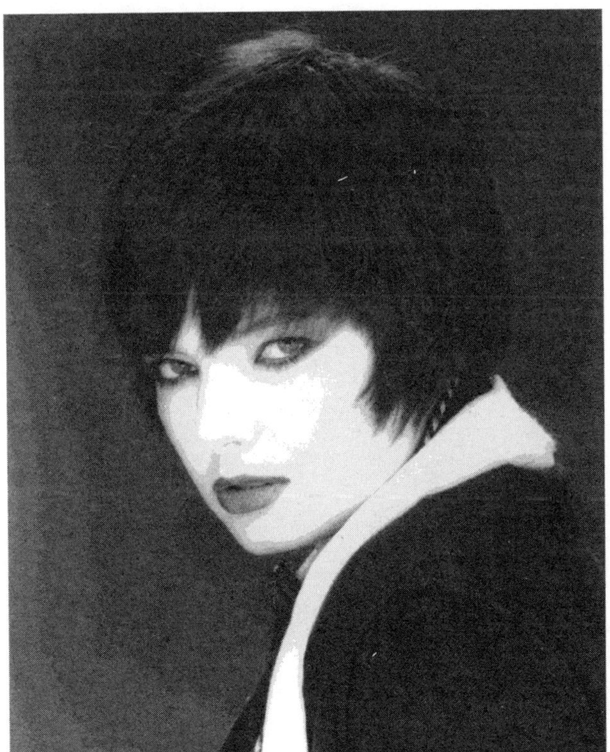

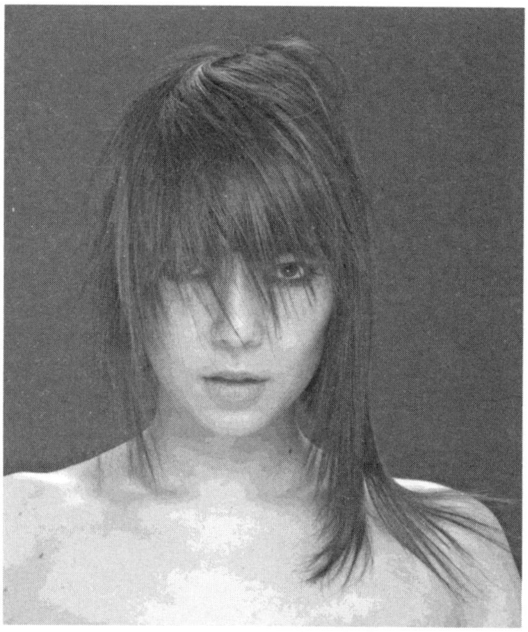

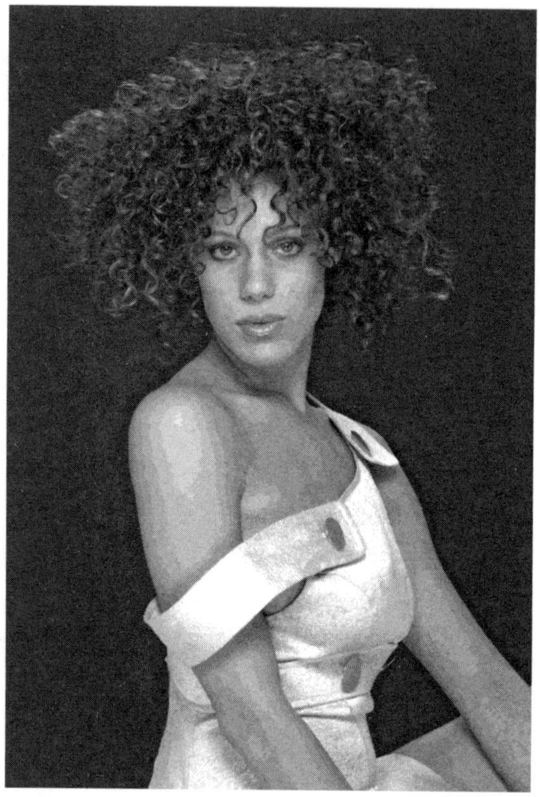

Top: Styled by Jason Edwards.
Right: Styled by Amy Edwards.

It's about the energy.

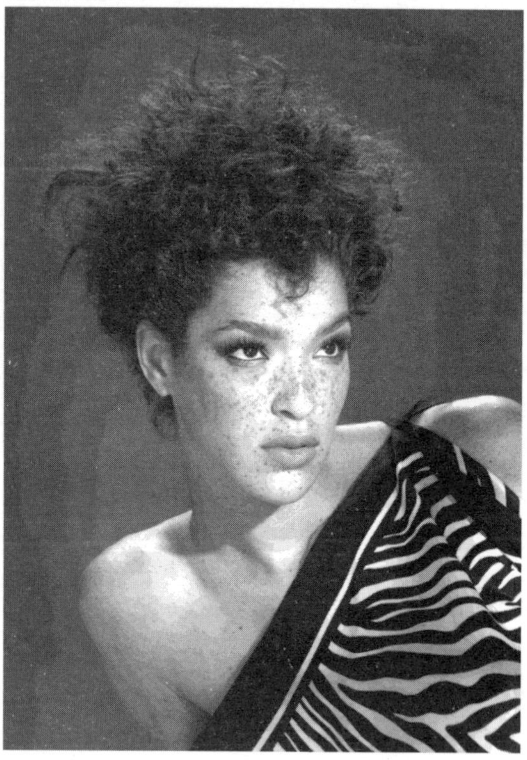

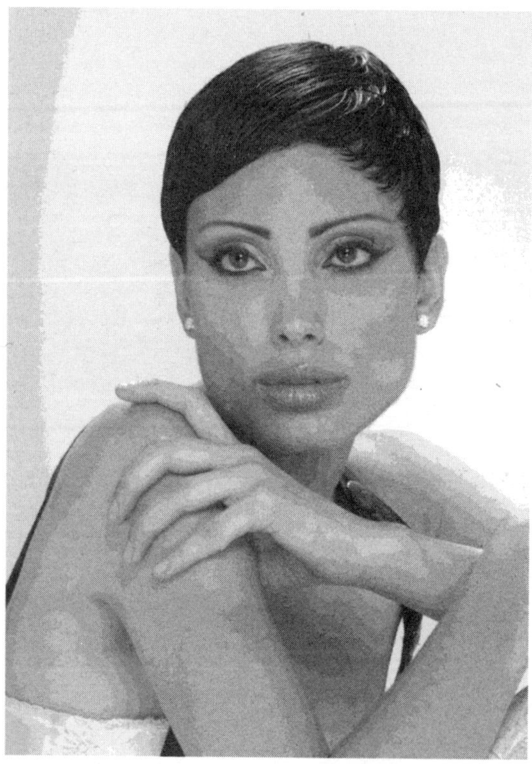

nine

By Shear Force

When I thought I'd lost Beverly Hills, I thought I'd lost everything. But I hadn't. I had just lost that space. Lisa did the most amazing thing. She had the guts to walk up to the landlord and negotiate a lower rent. Her logic was inescapable: If they didn't allow us to pay what we were currently paying, instead of raising the rent, we'd have to declare bankruptcy. And he worked with us for a little while. Ultimately, we ended up in a new space, a better space, and ultimately a better place. It was OK that Allen Edwards wasn't in Beverly Hills anymore. I hated the drive anyway.

When we lost Beverly Hills, Lisa stepped in. We had closed the body studio, and I was floundering. But ultimately Lisa was the key to getting me back on my feet, business-wise. She took over and started running the business. She became sort of the grim reaper and the person of reason all at once. She was the logical one; I was the nut bag. She's the best partner I've ever had.

Lisa had finally started to get better after having been diagnosed with Chronic Fatigue Syndrome. She had become a nutritionist after giving up the exercise studio. For six months she'd been at home, and during that time she got very involved with vitamins, minerals and herbs. She had been a medical assistant while she was in college and then went into cytology. After her illness and her subsequent recovery, nutrition became a very big deal. She even went back to school and got a degree in it. So it was a huge deal when I called her that fateful day.

"I think I need you to help me here," I said.

She was very quiet.

"Lisa?" I asked, not sure she had heard me.

"Did you hear what I said?" I asked.

Again, quiet.

"Because I, well, I think, if you could, I mean, if you want to, but I'd really like it, and I think I need your help."

She sighed.

"Is that a yes?" I asked tentatively, twirling my shears in my hand.

"My life is going to change. A lot," she said.

"I know," I said. "But I really need you." And I did. I'm not sure if I really knew what I was asking of her then. I wanted her to give up her job, doing something she absolutely loved, to come and bail my ass out. I realize now that it was a huge decision for her. That I was asking her to stop her life to help me.

"OK," she said. She told me later that she really felt like she had no choice. She had a life, but *we* had a life. And the salons were simply more important at the time. She understood that. The business was falling apart. She pulled it back together.

I don't know if I ever thanked her.

A sidebar: Lisa said recently that I didn't. I think she was kidding. But I also know that while she was working her ass off trying to get the business back on track, I had something else in mind: I wanted to redo my motorcycle. Made no sense. But I needed to do it. It was my way of dealing with defeat. By ignoring it.

"You want what?" Lisa asked, peering up at me from whatever paperwork was on her desk. I knew she loved me, but her eyes were daggers.

"Five thousand dollars," I said.

"I'm sorry?" she asked, pretending like she couldn't possibly have heard me correctly.

"Five thousand," I said, really quietly. "Dollars," I added even more quietly.

She stared at me. I looked down at my shoes.

She continued to stare. I knew she was thinking that I was nuts. Maybe I was. I decided to counter, and so I smiled.

She smiled, too, a little less enthusiastically than me. But she gave me the money.

I redid my bike. It motivated me to also re-do my career.

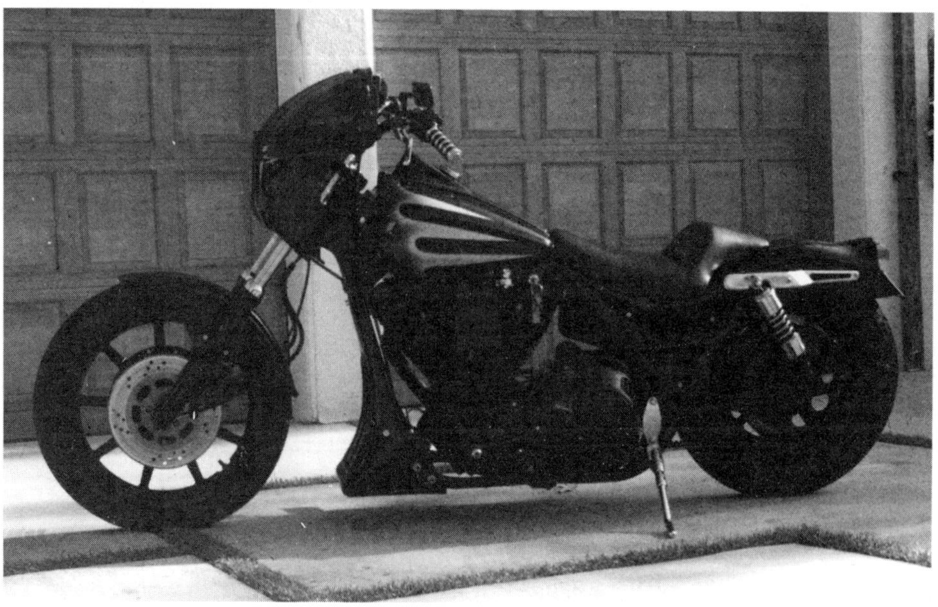

My beautiful baby.

I sold Beverly Hills to the guy who had been a thorn in my side for years. The guy who'd stolen all the hairdressers years before. He saved my ass. He ended up helping me. What goes around comes around.

The same day I had talked to a bankruptcy lawyer because I didn't know what to do about Beverly Hills, I met people who were building a brand-new shopping center on the corner of Laurel Canyon and Ventura Boulevard in Studio City. I knew I had to open a salon there. I convinced the owners to bankroll it and give me $300,000. I brought in a partner, Claudio Lazo. Eventually I ended up selling the salon to him (it's no longer called Allen Edwards. I don't make the same mistake twice).

I became an Aveda Concept Salon, something I now equate to a guy going to jail and suddenly becoming religious. I needed something to connect to, to turn me on, and I found it in Aveda.

Aveda, one of the original plant-based beauty companies and now owned by Estee Lauder, was the brainchild of a man named Horst Rachelbacker. He was a real character. Every year, he would put on this huge, three-day show in Minneapolis called Congress. He'd rent a theater for 5,000 people, invite five teams to perform and give out trophies. Hairdressers love trophies. Claudio and I were in the audience the year we opened Studio City.

"We'll be up on that stage next year," I whispered as I got up to go get a drink. I ran into Horst, who knew who I was, and he invited me to perform the following year. That was the jolt I needed.

I put together an hour and a half show for the next year. It was probably the best show I've ever done. I combined my vision of 1940s glam, romantic music and vintage dresses with geometric haircuts. Then I introduced the razor. I ended the show with me cutting hair like a lunatic, with girls in gas masks, dry ice and rockin' music. Standing ovation to follow. My daughter, Amy, was with me. It was her first big show, and she loved it.

That night, I remember going to Horst's home, where he had erected a huge tent. Actually, a huge Indian sweat lodge. He actually had indigenous Indians from the rainforest there, performing rituals, turning the temperature up. I said sweat lodge. Everyone was saying prayers, everyone was pouring sweat. It was a fucking nightmare.

We stayed an Aveda Concept Salon for the next year. Then I put my own makeup line in and Horst dropped me like a bad girlfriend. I became de-brainwashed. They sucked all the flower essence out of my brain and I was cured.

Onward.

We opened a salon in Brentwood to replace Beverly Hills. I've always loved Brentwood. It has a very East Coast flair. We kicked ass in the Woodland Hills salon.

Things were getting back on track.

It really started to turn around with Marcia Clark. The district attorney who was trying the case against O.J. Simpson had the unenviable task of trying the case on television. It was one of the first trials to be broadcast, which naturally left all parties open to criticism. It became about what people were wearing and how they looked. Were they tired? Had they been out drinking? What was really going on between Marcia and Chris (Christopher Darden, her co-counsel)?

And maybe most importantly: what the hell was going on with her hair?

She had this tight, mullet, poodle-like perm thing going on. It was old-fashioned and unattractive. One of my clients was in charge of publicity for the district attorney's office, and she realized that they were losing the war for public opinion. The public was more

infatuated with Johnny Cochran's antics (I mean, will any of us ever forget the line "If it doesn't fit, you must acquit"?) than with the facts.

To shake things up, something needed to shatter the buttoned-up, boring perception that the public had of Ms. Clark. Not that it would have made any difference in the outcome of the trial.

My client brought Marcia to me and sat her down in my chair.

"Do something, anything, make her dazzling," she said.

I talked to Marcia, a nice woman who was highly stressed and extremely tired. Getting her hair done seemed to be about the last thing on her mind.

A Good Hair Day

Prosecutor Marcia Clark Sheds Curls for a New Look

By TINA DAUNT
TIMES STAFF WRITER

He designed the 1970 "Charlie's Angels" mane of Farrah Fawcett and created the famous "frump" cut for Diane Keaton in the movie "Annie Hall."

Now Allen Edwards' scissors have once again sliced a place for him in the limelight—this time for the new hairstyle of O.J. Simpson prosecutor Marcia Clark, who returned to court Tuesday with a darker, straighter shag.

But even for a stylist who is accustomed to creating some of Hollywood's most buzzed-about styles, the attention stirred up by Clark's new do was a bit unnerving. By midafternoon, Edwards was inundated with more than 30 requests for interviews, from American Journal to ABC Radio News.

"I had a feeling people would react strongly," he said. "But not like this. It's just huge."

Clark almost looked like Sigourney Weaver, only more professional. Applause broke out among people waiting to enter the courtroom, including some reporters, when Clark walked past. "Get a life," laughed Clark, who obliged her admirers with a little pirouette.

The transformation started on Friday, when Clark called Edwards—who runs several salons in the Los Angeles area—to complain that she couldn't get her hair to curl properly. Edwards worked late Friday evening to fit Clark into his schedule at his Studio City salon.

At a cost of $150, Edwards trimmed and dyed Clark's hair a shade of auburn, replacing her trademark curls with a modified shag. On Tuesday morning, Edwards stopped at the prosecutor's home to blow-dry her new look—a service he provides for many of his famous clients, including Dustin Hoffman and Donna Mills.

"We can only do curl for so long and we both got tired of it," Edwards said of the prosecutor's new style. "It's her."

This is the second time Clark has changed her hairstyle in the globally televised O.J. Simpson murder trial, where much has been made of the appearances of the major players.

Last summer, Clark had her shoulder-length curls trimmed to the neckline—a hairstyle also created by Edwards, who offered his services to Clark after watching the prosecutor on television during the preliminary hearing.

"I hated her hair long," he said.

The latest change did not pass without a few remarks. Noted Deputy Dist. Atty. Christopher A. Darden: "Marcia told me that her hair was naturally curly."

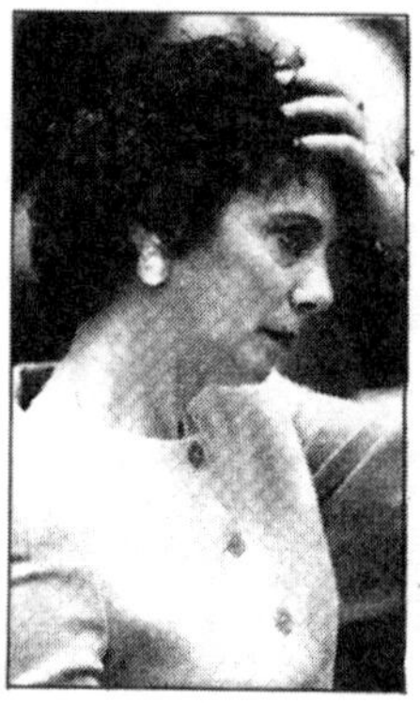
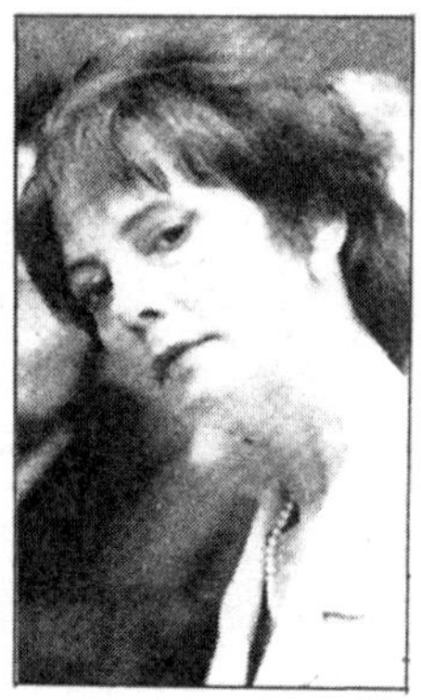

Pool Photos

At left, Marcia Clark in March as she questioned Brian (Kato) Kaelin, and in court on Tuesday.

The Marcia Clark phenomenon

Her perm was growing out. I cut off all the fuzz, shaped it, straightened it, and suddenly, she was a new woman. The papers covered it like it was the second coming. I was given credit for the transformation.

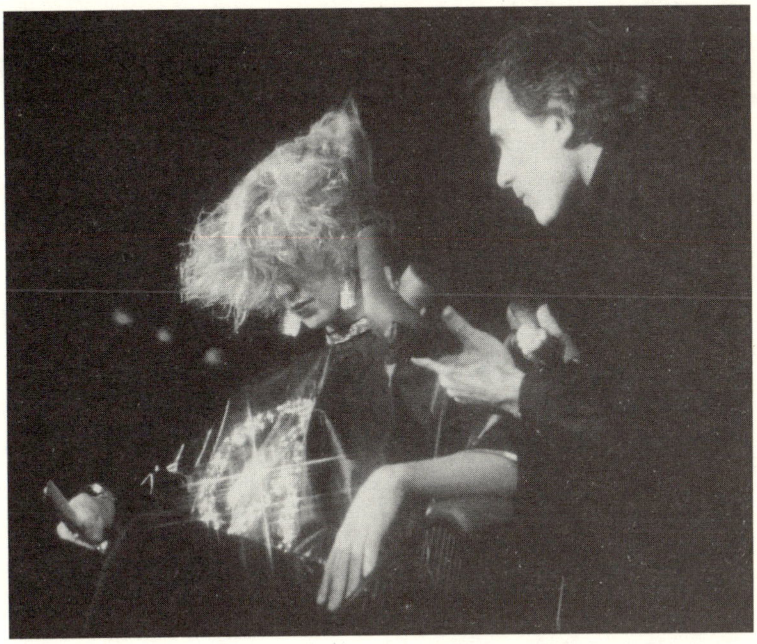

Rambo. With a blow dryer.

Suddenly I was back. My publicity machine was churning again. The phones in the salon started ringing.

Rambo with a blow dryer. A shear force of desire. Me, personified.

The press even started nosing around and rediscovered that it was me who had done the infamous "Farrah." *Extra* started following me around. Fame was knocking again. I was feeling good. I got invited to do the *Oprah* show. Oprah and I actually already had a relationship. It goes back to one of her first shows.

It happened early in the 1980s. She wasn't a huge star yet, not nearly what she was to become. But she was already on her way to being one of the most influential people in the entertainment industry. Hell, in the world. She had a real presence about her, a realness that I found disconcerting. I mean, I had been surrounded for years by the plastic bubble of Hollywood and Los Angeles. Chicago and Oprah Winfrey were definitely different.

Oprah was doing a makeover show. I was doing the hair portion of the makeovers, and I was very nervous. But it went very well, right up until the limo didn't show up to take me back to the airport. Oprah was going at the same time, and she noticed me standing outside the studio, hands shoved into my pockets, trying to look cool while I was freezing my ass off.

A black car pulled out from behind the studio and stopped. The window went down and her beautiful face popped out. She smiled.

"Who are you waiting for?" she asked.

"My ride," I said. "I'm supposed to catch a flight back to L.A. out of O'Hare. But I'm feeling a little stood up." I tried to smile. I must have succeeded.

"Well, I'm heading to O'Hare myself," she said. "Hop in. I'll give you a ride."

It took us an hour to get to the airport through rush hour traffic. She was charming, engaging, funny, and warm. I remember she took out a little velvet box and opened it to show me a beautiful ring, a diamond.

"Who would think that I would ever have something like this?" she said with a laugh.

Who would have thought she'd become who she has become today? I think I knew it then. I suspect she did, too.

I met her again, years later, at a spa in Ojai, California. I had my big mastiff dog with me and she was with her trainer. She recognized me and immediately came over to have a cup of coffee with Lisa and me. I think what impressed me most was that she remembered me.

Back to my comeback.

It was a Saturday, the salon was slammed, and I was leaving on a red-eye that night for Chicago. The phone rang and it was Farrah's manager. I was thinking, "Great, she wants me to do her hair again." He was thinking: "Nope." He ripped into me.

"Farrah's very upset," he said. "Farrah doesn't like that you're saying that you created her signature hairstyle. Farrah doesn't like it because Jose did it."

Jose, as in Jose Eber. He did do her hair, after the fact. After she got an ill-advised perm (not from me) and fried her hair.

So I was doing the Oprah show a couple of days later, and who walks in to also do the show but Jose Eber. I thought it might be uncomfortable, but evidently he didn't even know about the conversation.

I got introduced first:

"Ladies and gentlemen, I'd like to introduce the greatest hairdresser in the world, and the man who created the new look for Marcia Clark: Allen Edwards."

The crowd went wild.

I went on stage, the lights were shining, the audience was totally into it. I was doing hair, talking about the Marcia Clark. Jose wasn't doing any of the hair. His assistant was.

Then Oprah said, "Let's do one more look." Jose stepped up and talked about it.

We were very professional. Hell, I like Jose. Always have. We have a camaraderie.

Time went by, and then the *Charlie's Angels* movie came out and I was getting even more press, especially about the Farrah. Once again, she was furious and sent her lawyer to see me. He threatened to sue, so I sent the picture of Farrah and me. She wanted Jose to have the credit because they were personal friends. I think she even bought him his first hat like the one he wears all the time.

But no matter how hard she tried, the Farrah cut was then and remains mine. I'm fine with that.

The lesson I learned through all of this was simple: never give up. Always focus on the future. Don't wallow in regret. Use that get-out-of-jail card any way you can in order to pick up the shards of your life, glue them back together and make something brand new.

I was riding high in the 1970s. In the '80s, things started crashing down around me, culminating in my losing my partners and my salons. In the '90s, I roared back. My salons are #4 on *Salon City* magazine's "Hot 100 Salons in America." And I've never looked behind me to see where I've been.

After the Marcia Clark thing, I jumped on my motorcycle. I rode out to Mulholland Highway and cruised. The sun was setting, the air was cool, and the sky was a pale shade of its former daytime self. The engine vibrated beneath me and the power propelled me forward. The force of it was exhilarating and my body felt electrified.

As I drove along, obeying the speed limit, I reflected on my life. I'm not for reflection usually, but this time was different. Something about making my way back from the brink of financial disaster was strangely freeing. I felt like I could accomplish anything after that. On my bike that day, I couldn't think of a thing I needed to accomplish.

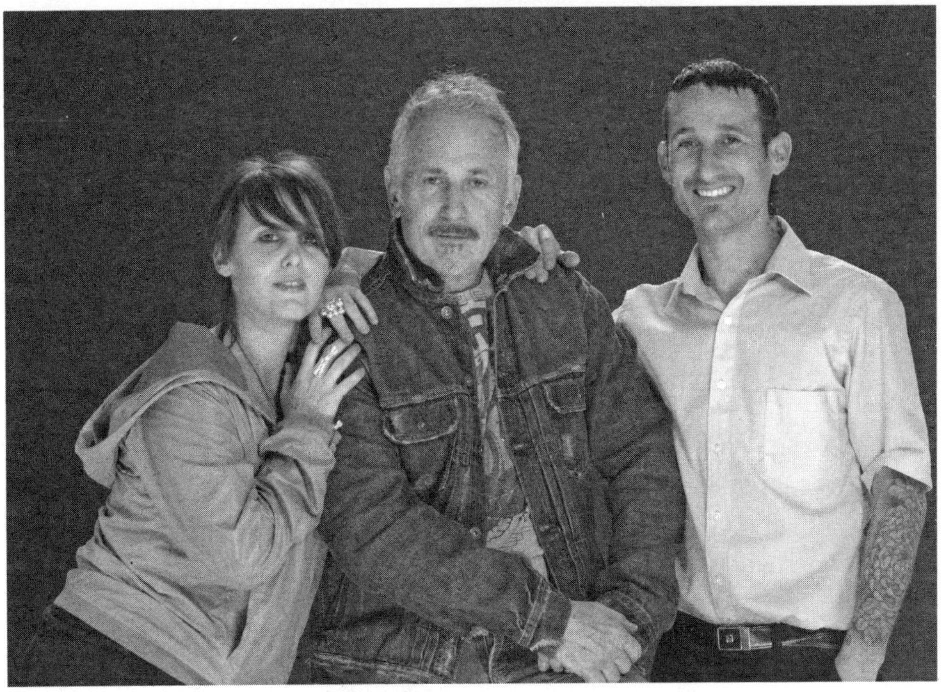

My kids, Amy and Jason.

Lisa and I have had an interesting life together, once we got together. We raised her two kids, Megan and Samantha, and my two kids, Amy and Jason.

Both of my kids have become hairdressers. Jason had a rough start as a teen. To help him get on track, I sent him to Israel and he lived on a kibbutz for two years, which he loved. Today, he's a loving, responsible hairdresser who loves family and loves life. He looks a little like Sean Penn. He's got an amazing talent. He looks at hairdressing as art, just like I do. I feel Jason is on his way to being the next Allen Edwards. Recently, he was written up on the front page of the *Los Angeles Times* Style section, and his PR machine is kicking in. I finally found a replacement. His next step is to own his own salon and enter the world of stress. (Let the good times begin.)

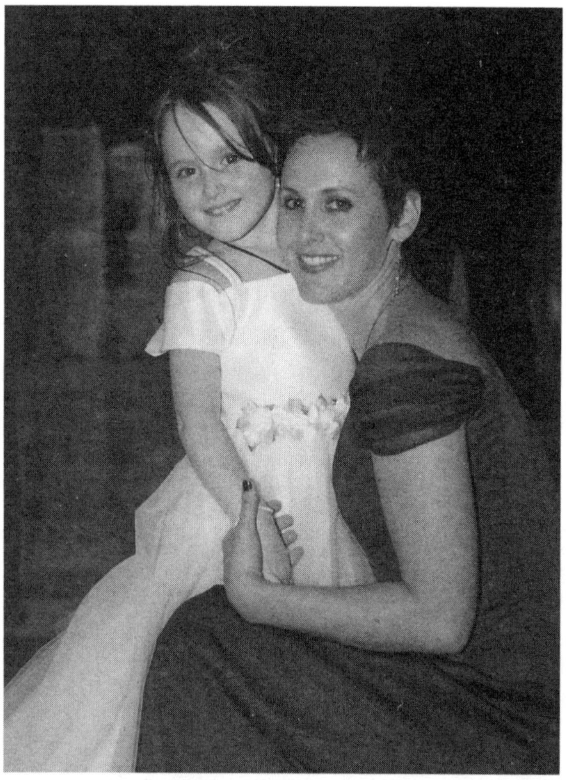

My daughter and my granddaughter.

Amy got married, had a child, got divorced. She has her own style, very independent, very artistic. Very driven. Very like me. She used to go to my shows when she was younger, and she just absorbed it all. She was even on stage with me a couple of times. She's just an amazing talent. She also pursued a show career. She's currently a top platform artist for Wella. My granddaughter's name is Benny Goodman. Amy's artistic talents are taking her in many directions, including writing her own book about training assistants.

Both of Lisa's daughters have found their place in the world. Along with being close with Lisa and their dad (and me), they're also very close with each other as well.

Megan is married. Just had a baby, a little boy named Ethan. She has worked in the salon in the past, in the office. She now works with her husband, James.

Samantha is an MFCC therapist, specializing in art therapy. She also has a little boy named Jacob. We call him Jake. Her husband, Jeff Shapiro, is a film producer and owns a camera company called Worldwide Digital Services.

Lisa's ex-husband, Phil, and I have a great relationship. Fran is still around, somewhere. As love goes, everyone finds his or her mate. Fran found hers in a lawyer, Phil found his in an event coordinator. I found my dancer. And my dancer found me: Allen Edward Goldstein.

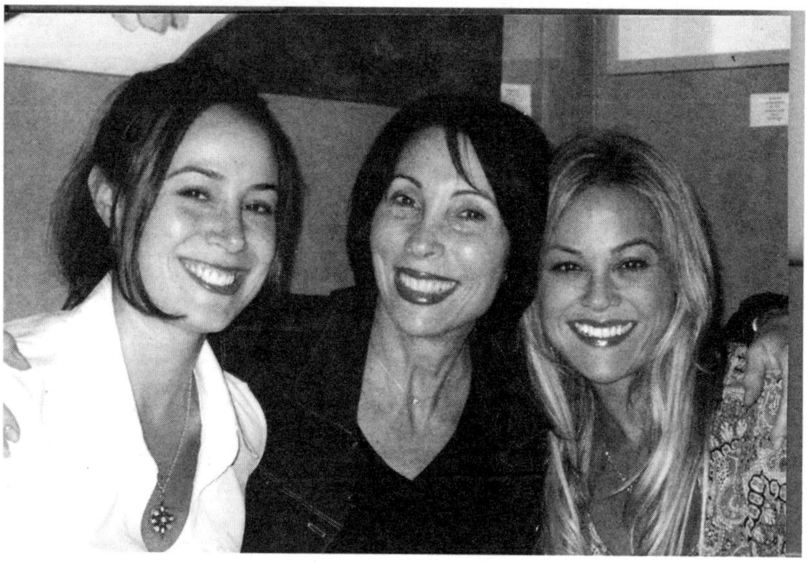

Megan, Lisa and Samantha.

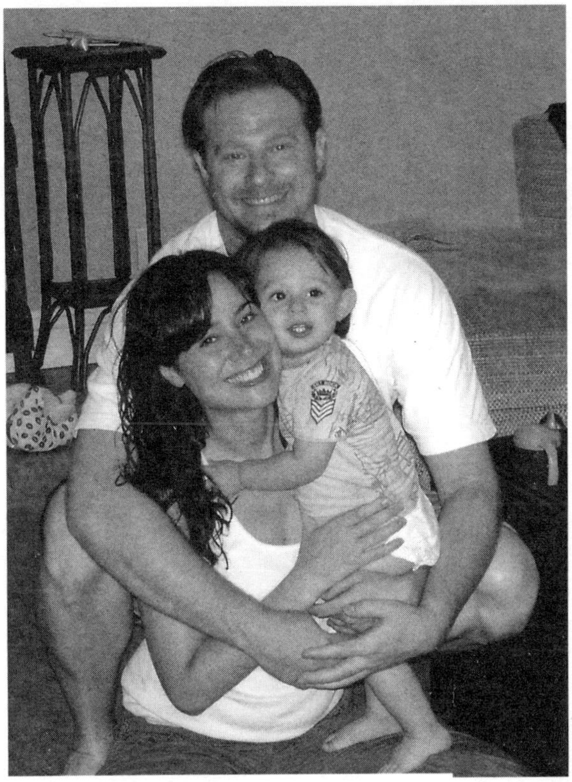

Sam and Jeff with Jake.

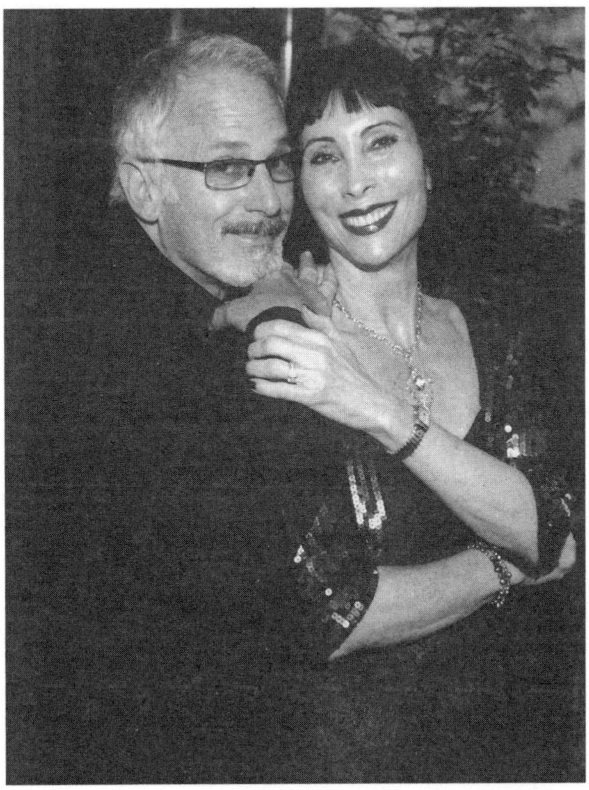

Lisa and me today.

Reflections

wrapping it all up

The View from Here

An image-maker's thoughts on the future

It's funny. I sit here, at the end of this book, thinking back on these episodes in my life. And here's what I know. The 1970s were about the cliché: sex, drugs and rock 'n roll. It was a decade devoted to bad fashion, the perfect hair flip, and getting laid. When the '70s began, I was 19 years old. My hormones were screaming. I would drive down the street looking for girls. Eventually I had a list of girls I could call so I could stop by after work and get laid. It was like a real life porno movie.

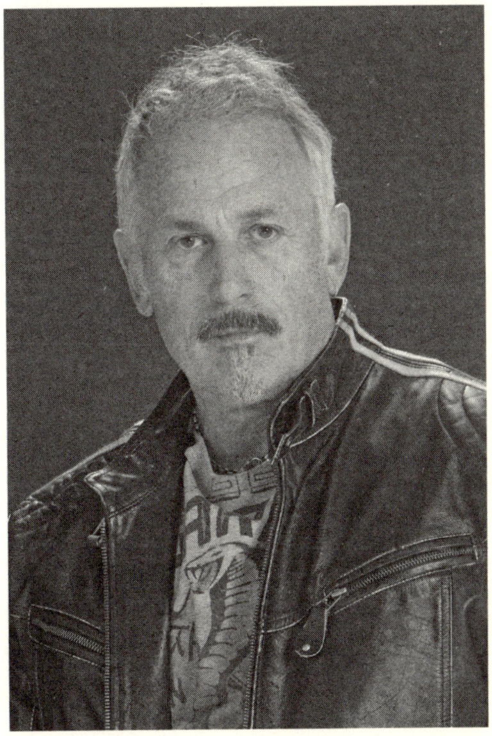

In the '80s, it was all about my television career taking off. On the other hand, the AIDS epidemic hit and I lost a lot of close friends. I also got divorced and my business started falling apart. That's when the world—my world—came to a screeching halt.

The '90s were about coming back. Getting my life back on track, retaking my name, recharging my career.

It's because of all of this, because of everything I've lived through, that I now know this: love is what's most important, and that positivity gives you power. (Yeah, that's a word I made up.) We can fool around our whole lives, but that's just sex, not love. None of that matters.

I know that it's important to feel accomplished. It started for me when I was eight years old, playing the trumpet. I knew that I could feel as if I'd done something by learning to play a song, by standing in front of a crowd and performing, by not stuttering. That sense of accomplishment has been with me ever since. Hell, it might have been with me before I discovered that horn.

I still have that trumpet, and I look at it sometimes. I pull it down from the shelf and blow off the dust. I open the case and I see that the brass has tarnished. I've actually started to play again. My passion for it has come back.

It reminds me that taking chances is always a good thing. It's also scary. But if you take a chance, just imagine what you might create.

You know, in the movie *Evan Almighty*, Morgan Freeman says something to this effect: God can't make you creative, but he can give you the opportunity to be creative. It's all about opportunity. It's about the validation, and yeah, it's a little about the money. Hey, I'm nothing if not honest. You know that about me by now.

After reading this, you either think I'm an idiot, an egomaniac, or a combination. That's OK. I'm probably a little bit of both. I'm also a survivor. I'm a hairdresser. An entrepreneur. A husband. A father. A lover.

I can even be a fighter. Recently I cut this girl's hair and she didn't like it. Something that doesn't happen all that often. She came back at the end of the day with her boyfriend. Her 30-year-old boyfriend who was about 9 feet tall. He wanted to know what my problem was when I cut her hair.

"She's your problem, man, not mine," I said. He didn't like it. Wonder why.

He stepped into my face. Nose to nose. Well, maybe not nose-to-nose since he was about a foot taller. I stood there for a minute, eyes blazing, breath snorting, hair standing on end.

"If you want to go with me, fucker, I'll take you down right now," I hissed. Then I pushed him into the mirror.

He walked away, but before he got out the door, he stopped and turned. I'm standing there all big and bad.

"Faggot," he said and pushed out into the night.

Wow. Good one. Like I'd never heard THAT before. When I told Lisa about it later that night she just shook her head and said: "I'd expect nothing less from you. But you're either going to end up in the hospital or in jail."

No jail for me. I play Monopoly, remember?

I'm constantly creating, even today. Reinventing and being reborn. It has nothing to do with age, even though the age factor comes into play big time in the beauty industry (and in the entertainment industry. I'm screwed both ways). Interestingly, my age and my experience are giving me a tremendous amount of credibility.

It's the same in entertainment. When you're great, you're great no matter how old you are. It's like Anthony Hopkins and Sean Connery. Older actors want—love—to keep working just like I do, but they have to reinvent themselves. They have to be smart enough to take a different type of part. And when they do, their lives continue to be full and rewarding. People in the arts need to stay in touch with their artistic side. People who aren't in the arts need to stay in touch with whatever floats their boat. Age has nothing to do with it. It's just a state of mind. Nothing more and a lot less.

Embrace where you are at any time. I do, I am. It's about making life as full and rewarding as possible. You have to take opportunities when they come. Don't be afraid, even when you are. Pretend. It's easier than you might think. Opportunity can make you feel better about what you're doing, no matter what job you have. If you own a gas station and you have the opportunity to expand the station into a car wash and detail shop, go for it.

Go for it.

No matter what you do, there's opportunity to do more, do better.

My fear of failure has always pushed me in the opposite direction, fighting not to fail and to feel success. And yet, I've had some huge failures. But I don't dwell on the failure. If you think you're a loser, you're no good. If you think you're a success, you will be. I really believe that. I've LIVED that. And I'm happier than ever. I have new goals. Life's different. Life's good.

Now it's about teaching my grandkids how to water-ski, how to have fun, how there's no such thing as failing.

In the end, I think that life is like a big Monopoly game. We're all going to end up at the end of the board. We'll either have lots of hotels and property—and money—or we'll be dead broke. But ultimately it's about how you played the game. It's about how full your life is. That's what really matters. Because you never know where the game is going to take you. It's all about the opportunity. It doesn't matter if you land on Park Place and buy it. It matters that you knew about Park Place to begin with. (It also matters that you avoid jail at all costs.)

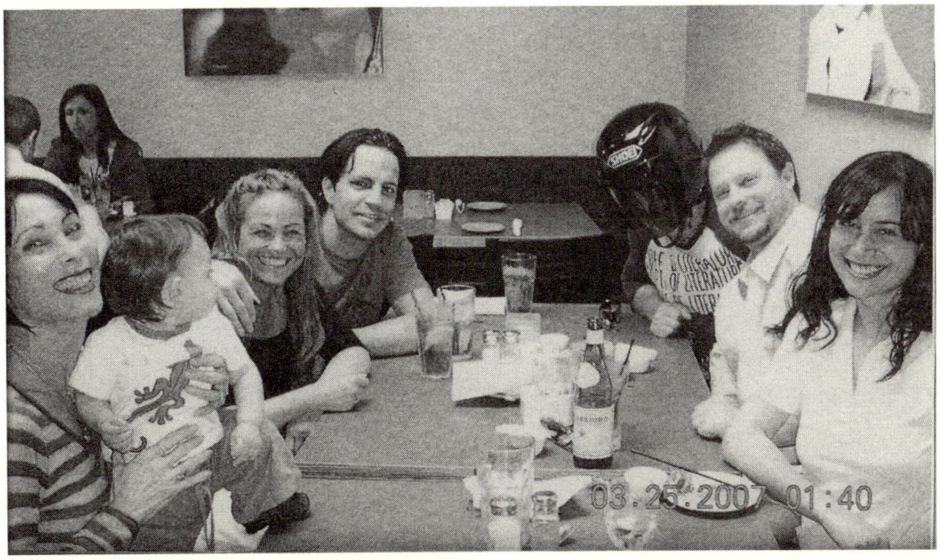

The family. Me, in the helmet. Always wear protection.

I spent a lot of time in gestalt therapy. I've learned not to dwell on the past because I can't change it. I deal with the reality I have, and that reality is pretty damned good. This is the best time in my life. A new game is just beginning. Just give me the dice and watch me roll.

I can't wait to see where I land.

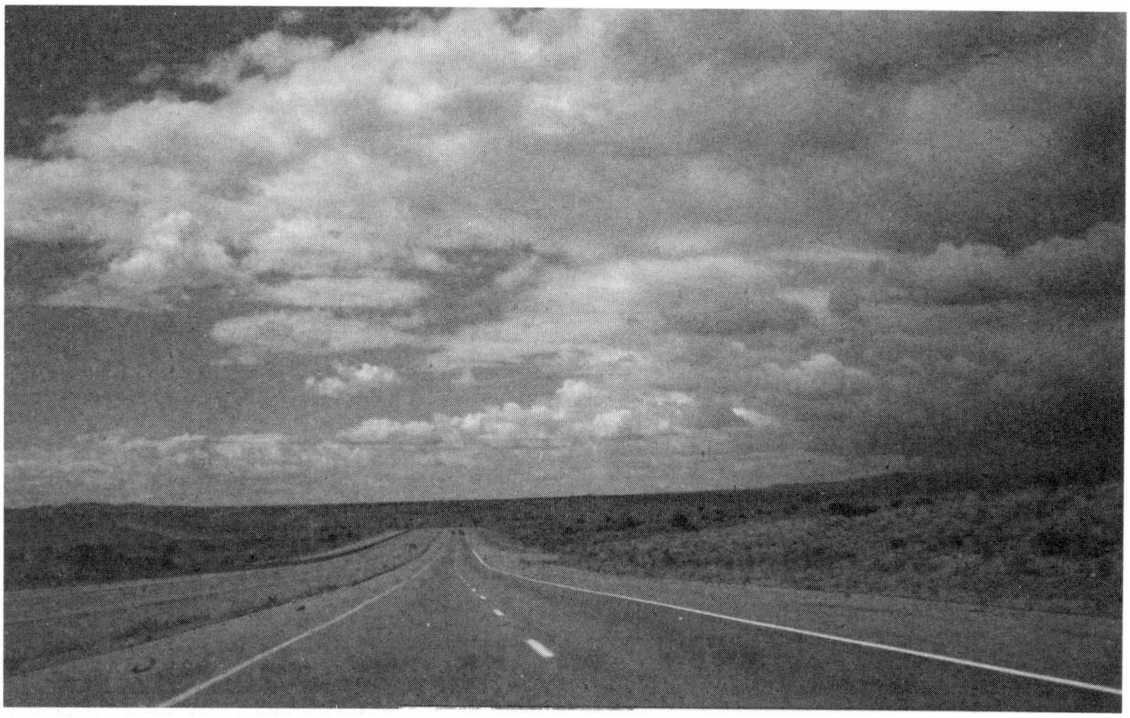